# Skin Secrets

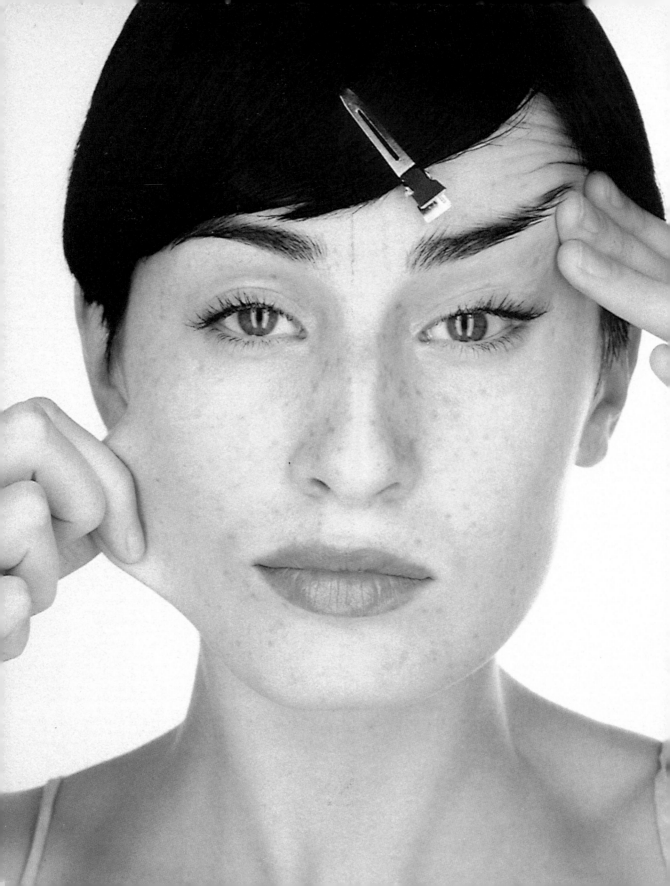

# Skin Secrets

## The Medical Facts versus the Beauty Fiction

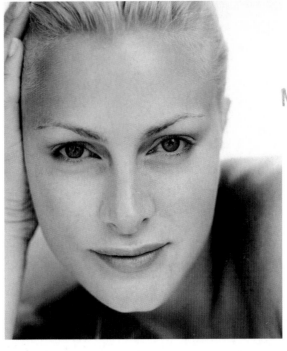

Professor Nicholas Lowe MD • Polly Sellar

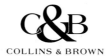

C&B

COLLINS & BROWN

Acknowledgements

There have been many scientific and clinical advances in understanding and treating ageing, damaged and diseased skin. Many of these advances have resulted from the painstaking research conducted by many dermatologist colleagues and research scientists. Some of the relevant knowledge is summarized in our book. We are very grateful for it.

My especial thanks to my wife Pam and daughters Nichola and Philippa. *Professor Nicholas Lowe* MD

My especial thanks to Dr Daniel Maes, (vice president of research and development at Estee Lauder) and Dr Hugh Rushton PhD, to *Vogue* readers whose phone calls over the years provided the impetus for this book, and to my husband, Jono. *Polly Sellar*

Our joint thanks to our publishers and editors – Cindy Richards, Liz Dean and Mary Lambert – for their support and guidance, and to our agent, Maggie Pearlstine

First published in Great Britain in 1999
by Collins & Brown Limited, London House
Great Eastern Wharf, Parkgate Road
London SW11 4NQ

Distributed in the United States and Canada by Sterling Publishing Co,
387 Park Avenue South, New York, NY 10016, USA

A CIP catalogue record of this book is available from the British Library.

ISBN 1-85585-665-4

9 8 7 6 5 4 3 2 1

NOV 5 1999

Editor: Mary Lambert
Design: XAB Design

Reproduction by: Classic Scan, Singapore
Printed and bound in Portugal by Printer Portuguesa

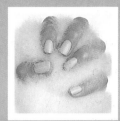 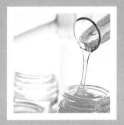 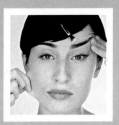

# contents

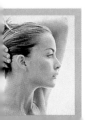

# introduction

Not so very long ago, the way our skin looked and aged was thought to be a matter of whether or not we'd inherited 'good skin' genes. Then, cosmetic scientists formulated sweet-smelling concoctions that even their makers famously dubbed 'hope in a jar', dermatologists managed

## Retinoids can temporarily reverse the ageing process and lasers can dramatically alter the look of time-worn skin

skin diseases, and for those who wanted to turn back time, surgery was the only option.

But where once drugs treated skin disease and cosmetics merely moisturised, now the line between the two is blurring. Today, the truly 'anti-ageing' cream is no longer the holy grail of cosmetic science, but a prescribable option. The ageing process itself is no longer an inevitability but something that happens 'prematurely'. And Instead of having to choose between growing

old gracefully and submitting to the scalpel, we now have quick-fix wrinkle fillers and rapid-fire skin resurfacing lasers.

The seachange came when it was realised that our skin is not the inert, impenetrable barrier we once thought it, and that the sun, and not natural ageing process is the blame for most of the lines and wrinkles, dark spots and thread veins that define the older face. As a result, the last decade has seen a multitude of new skin-treating creams, drugs and devices pouring onto the cosmetic and healthcare markets. Broad spectrum sun-filtering day creams can now help slow the ageing process, topically applied retinoids can temporarily reverse it, and resurfacing lasers can dramatically alter the look of time-worn skin.

But as the possibilities proliferate, so too, does the confusion. What can AHAs do? Is laser resurfacing safe? How can a vitamin-A derivative drug smooth sun-worn skin? But how can the average skin cream consumer know the answers to these questions if the basics are still in question? Should cleanser be tissued or rinsed off? How often should you exfoliate? Is SPF15 every day really necessary? This book will answer all these questions and more. It brings together the latest and the basics – the low-down on the newest laser procedures and advice on good, scientifically-sound daily skincare regime.

Some books tell you that great skin comes courtesy of a DIY avocado and mayonnaise face pack. Some books insist you can simply eat yourself beautiful. There is even one insisting you think yourself beautiful. This book gives you the medical facts about how to have, and to hold, a great, clear, young-looking skin. The following chapters reveal everything that the modern cosmetic, dermatologist now knows about what skin needs to look its glowing, radiant best. It includes lay translations of the latest empirical information borne out of clinical trials, published in dermatological journals, presented at international conferences, and subjected to the scrutiny of medical peers. It has been written to help you make sense of what's really going on in a rapidly changing, and increasingly baffling, beauty industry, to assist you in sorting what's possible from what's implausible, to allow you to sift the medical facts

of skincare matters from the beauty fiction. It offers the sort of independent advice that in a ferociously competitive skincare market, and increasingly competitive skin clinic market, is so hard to come by.

The information contained in *Skin Secrets* will put you, the preyed-upon skincare consumer back in the driving seat. You will know what your skin needs and why. You will be able to make informed choices about what to buy, how much to spend, and when to consult a dermatologist. You will know what skin creams can and can't do, and if you want radical results, what options are available and where to go for them. For instance, once you have read Chapter 2 you should be able to walk up to any cosmetic counter and instead of asking the consultant, 'What should I be using?' you will be able to say, 'This is what I should be using. What do you have that fits the bill?' Once you've read Chapter 3, you will know why SPF15 sunscreens, not diamonds, are a girl's best friend. And if, or when, the time comes that you think you need more than over-the-counter creams have to offer, Chapters 6–8 will spell out what realistic results you can expect from cosmeceuticals, wrinkle fillers, chemical peels and laser rejuvenation.

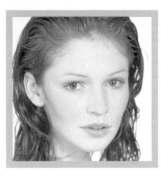
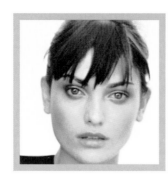
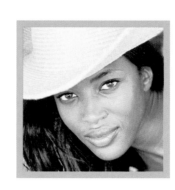

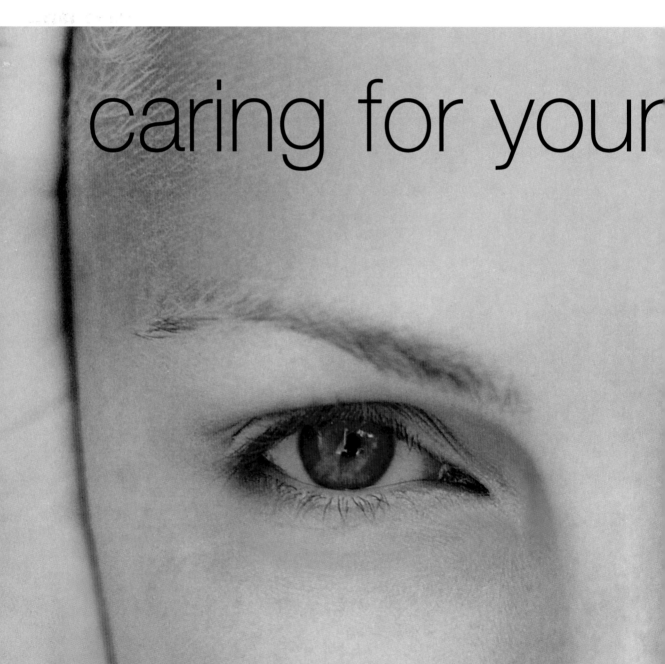

caring for your

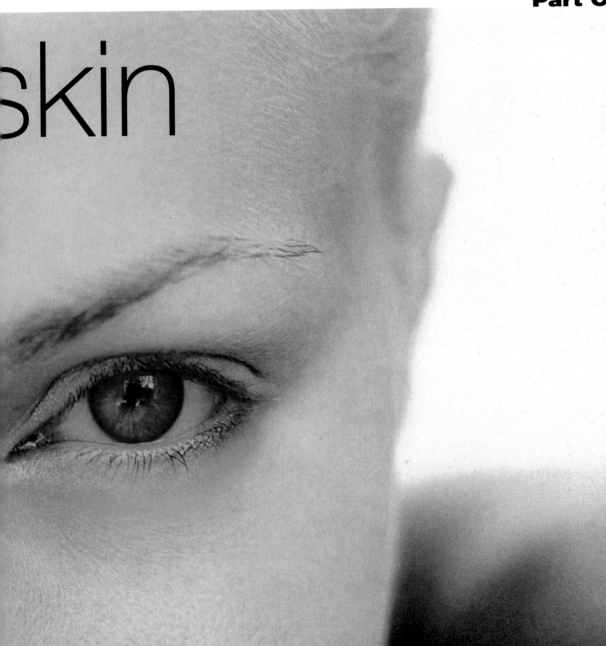

# skin

# 1

## UNDER YOUR SKIN

**You are covered in it – in fact about 2 sq metres (2¹/₂ sq yd) of it. It's only about 4 mm (¹/₈ in) at its thickest, on the soles of your feet, but weighs in total about 4 kg (9 lbs), or 7 per cent of your total body weight.**

# your skin

protects your internal organs, lets your body breathe, and helps you resist bacteria and infection. It is not, however, simply an inert, squishy envelope which keeps all the really vital bits of your body together: your skin is, in fact, itself an organ. At its most basic level, it protects us but, like our other vital organs, it

## Your skin is not, however, simply an inert, squishy envelope which keeps all the really vital bits of your body together.

performs a number of exchange functions, absorbing what's useful to us and secreting what is damaging. However, unlike your other organs, your skin is on permanent display. It is, literally and metaphorically, the face you show to the world. How our skin functions is of almost no day-to-day concern, not least because, for most of us, it does its job perfectly and unremarkably. The pressing concern most of us have is more superficial; we care about how our skin looks.

A clear, smooth, glowingly healthy complexion is the ideal that we all seek. Some of us are lucky enough to have it naturally, others have

to actively pursue it. Whether you are trying to improve your complexion or just keep the one you've got, you'll be better able to do so by understanding more of how your skin works, what it's made up of, and what is actually happening when it starts to wrinkle or develop spots.

## Your skin's function

Your skin is your protective barrier to harmful external substances such as bacteria, foreign bodies, chemicals and UV light. It also helps to retain your water electrolytes and other essential body fluids.

Skin is your body's heat regulator, cooling you with sweat when hot, and restricting the blood supply to the extremities when it is cold. And by sending out pain signals, it helps safeguard you from potentially fatal injury.

## Your skin's construction

Your skin is made up of three distinct layers: the epidermis (top layer), the dermis (the middle layer) and the subcutis (the bottom layer).

### The epidermis

This is the highly metabolically active top layer in which skin cells and pigment are 'manufactured'. The horny outer layer is the stratum corneum.

# Chapter One

From their place of origin in the lower epidermis, new cells go on a month-long journey towards the surface. For the first two weeks, as they travel through the 'living' epidermis, these cells are round, plump and with a fully functioning nucleus. But as they near the summit, they shrivel and flatten out, the nucleus begins to break down and they fill with a tough protein called keratin. This process is called cornification. By the time the cells reach the surface they are flat, scaly, desiccated versions of their former selves. And as such, they are perfectly poised to fulfill their final role – that of protecting you from the outside world.

What you see when you look at your skin is the stratum corneum. It is made up from between 18 to 23 layers of these flat dry skin cells cemented together into a defensive wall by a cocktail of fatty compounds such as lipids, peptides, ceramides and sebum. The primary function of any skincare regime is to keep this wall as solid as possible (see Chapter 2). It is your best bet for great looking, problem-free skin. Unfortunately, however, the stratum corneum is relatively easily damaged – by the sun's rays (see Chapter 3) and also by the detergents and surfactants we use for cleansing (see Chapter 2).

As new cells push up to the skin's surface from beneath, the dead scaly ones are invisibly sloughed off to form dust (or fodder for the dust mite). In your lifetime, you will make and lose on average several kg of skin. The process of shedding skin is called desquamation.

**beauty spot**

- The outer layer of a premature baby's skin is underdeveloped and incapable of regulating body temperature

- A baby's skin doesn't become a fully effective barrier until full thickness occurs at about six months. It is, therefore, important to use specifically formulated bath products for this very sensitive skin, and to keep babies shaded from the sun.

Also contained in the epidermis are the spidery-shaped melanocytes, which produce the skin's natural pigment, melanin. Whatever our colouring or race, we all have a similar number of melanocytes. The difference lies in the amount of melanin each produces. Melanin is a dark treacley substance that is manufactured in response to ultraviolet assault. It migrates into individual cells to form a physical umbrella over the nucleus to protect it against sun damage. It is also a fabulously potent neutralizer of skin-ageing free radicals (see page 20).

The more melanin you produce, the darker your skin and the better protected it is from ultraviolet damage. Very pale skin produces almost no melanin, or if it does, it tends to be a poor-quality variety (phaeomelanin) which often coagulates into all but useless clumps, or freckles. Black skin, on the other hand, produces copious amounts of really useful, and evenly distributed eumelanin. Nevertheless, even the darkest black skins are estimated to offer a natural sun protection factor (SPF) of only about 10. (For more on melanin and its role in skin protection, see Chapter 3.)

## The dermis

This middle layer is deep and spongy containing collagen and elastin which acts like a supportive, elastic mattress to the epidermis. Up to 3 mm (⅛) in thick, the dermis is your skin's main foundation. It is an unseen supportive network that forms a firm resilent basis for what sits on top. About 95 per cent of the dermis is made up of collagen, the body's wondrous shock asborber – found everywhere in the body from skin and muscles to tendons and cartilage.

Elastin makes up about 3 per cent of the dermis. As its name implies, it is a stretchy substance, its fibres arranged into springy coils which enables the skin to snap back into place after moving or being pulled.

Hair follicles sit in the depths of the dermis along with sebaceous (or oil) glands and sweat glands. Sebaceous glands are attached alongside the hair follicle, feeding off the same blood supply and using the hair shaft as a natural passageway to get sebum, the skin's natural oil, up to the surface where it spreads out to form a good barrier against moisture loss. Sweat glands have a dual role: firstly, they work to extract excess salts and other toxins, using water to wash them away. Secondly, they help lower a hot body's temperature by releasing liquid onto the skin which evaporates and reduces the heat. A variety of receptor corpuscles are situated in the dermis and are responsible for sensation – touch, vibration, pressure and warm and cold feelings.

The dermis supports and feeds the epidermis with all the nutrients, vitamins and chemicals it needs to produce an effective barrier. It runs the skin's repair, immune and sensory systems, and produces sebum and sweat. It also protects your vital organs from UV damage and injury.

### The subcutis

Consisting mainly of fat cells interspersed with blood vessels, bundles of nerve fibres and some fingers of muscle fibre, the subcutis acts as a protective cushion for what lies above and below. It also supports the blood vessels and muscle and nerve fibres. Its depth, not surprisingly, depends on how fat you are; it may be several centimetres deeper over your buttocks while over the eyelids it may be just a few cells thick.

### As good as it gets

Frustratingly, this happy state of affairs (see Boxes 1–5 below) when your skin glows with youthful clarity and vigour and requires nothing from you in return, persists only as long as you remain oblivious of it – from the age of six months through until the onset of puberty. However, the good news is that there is now an infinitely greater understanding of how and why the skin ages and what can be done to preserve its youthful condition. Keeping your skin looking as fantastic at 46 as it did at six may not be the sinecure it once was, but with careful preventive measures, and a few of the really effective cures currently becoming available, great-looking skin can be yours at any age.

## How Skin Should Be
**When your skin is functioning at its best from 6 months to puberty:**

**1** **The stratum corneum** is a smooth, tight wall of neat cells bound together by slippery ceramides and sebum – enough to keep the skin moist and supple, but not so much as to cause pore blockages and spots. Water is locked behind this wall and the passage of foreign invaders is blocked. The desquamation process is efficient with dead skin cells being easily and evenly shed so that your complexion looks and feels smooth.

**2** **Your skin tone** is bright because the fine, clear stratum corneum allows blood and colour to glow from below.

**3** **The epidermis** makes copious numbers of perfect new skin cells, and melanin is evenly distributed throughout it.

**4** **Any damage done** to the skin at this stage is quickly repaired: bits of damaged DNA are taken out and replacement parts are rapidly dispatched while any wounds are hastily repaired.

**5** **Your subcutis** is plump and even, giving your face and body the smooth, even contours of youth.

13

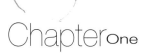

# Chapter One

## Through the ages – how your skin changes

**All skin goes through a natural ageing process through the decades. Some of the changes are inevitable; others, happily, are perfectly preventable.**

### In your teens

Up until puberty, your skin should generally look bright and clear. But already the effects of ultraviolet light are even being indelibly etched onto your epidermal blueprint, but the damage won't become apparent for some years yet – if at all – provided you start wearing SPF15 every day.

As adolescence strikes, however, those pesky hormones which are responsible for the dramatic changes throughout your body, also boost the production of the natural skin oil, sebum.

become a real worry, consult a dermatologist for specialist acne treatment. (See also Chapter 6).

Despite the increased oil and subsequent spots, cell generation is still running at its all time high of about a 28-day turnover during your teens. The dermis is still plump, and its collagen and elastin are still perfectly cross linked and coiled.

### In your 20s

Your twenties should be another reasonably stable time for your skin. By now any teenage

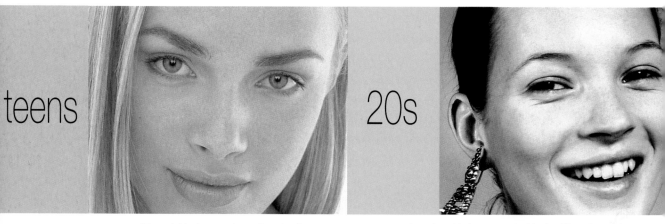

teens

20s

Thought to be a primeval protective response to impending adulthood, a more negative side-effect of this increased oil is the dreaded spots.

As the sebum flows freely from the sebaceous glands, dead skin cells adhere to it and the skin and hair pores get blocked up. An uninfected blocked pore is a blackhead, while ones infected with bacteria become red raised pimples or whiteheads. You can help prevent spots by washing your face with specialist over-the-counter washes (look for ones containing salicylic acid or benzoylperoxide), but if the spots

spots should have subsided. (If not seek specialist treatment – see Chapter 6.)

You probably won't have any visible facial lines, but if you look in the mirror as you talk, laugh or scowl you will see where your 'expression' lines will form. Your stratum corneum may be slightly less even and marginally thicker as dead skin cells aren't being shed quite as successfully. However, your epidermis is still plump and should hold up well – provided you keep it well protected. Turnover of new cells, however, may have slowed slightly from its 28-day peak.

If you are wearing sun-filtering day creams your skin is protected, but if not it is in your dermis that the greatest changes are taking place. The daily wear-and-tear wrought by UVA radiation could now be taking the bounce and spring out of your collagen bundles and elastin coils. Production of collagen is slowing, the bundles are less uniformly cross linked, elastin coils less tightly sprung.

### In your 30s

Your complexion starts to lose some of its youthful bloom as cell turnover slows and the stratum corneum fills with desiccated cells. A cosmetic alpha hydroxy acid (AHA) preparation (see Chapter 2) or a stronger dermatologist-prescribed one (see Chapter 7) will soon get you glowing again.

frown, the fat of the subcutis is pushed into trenches. Gradually, it becomes less likely to return to its original smooth shape – and the dreaded wrinkles start to form. However, they are a good few years away yet and the way that cosmetic dermatology is advancing there will be even more options for reducing wrinkles than already exist (see Chapters 7–9).

### In your 40s

Sebum production is markedly reduced, which is a boon for people with oily skins. If your skin was always normal to dry, you will benefit from some of the highly efficient moisturizers that are now available. A good moisturizer can do wonders to plump up fine dry lines and generally make your

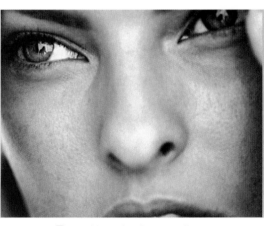

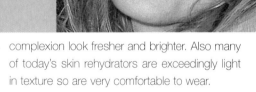

The epidermal cells are suffering more mutations picked up through environmental damage, although signs of this damage may not yet be visible. If you haven't worn them yet, then starting to use high SPF day creams now will not only keep any further deterioration at bay, but can actually give your skin a chance to do some repair work.

Your dermis is beginning to lose some of its volume and bounce: collagen fibres are no longer as efficiently meshed and the elastin coils aren't quite as tight. Moreover, as you smile and

complexion look fresher and brighter. Also many of today's skin rehydrators are exceedingly light in texture so are very comfortable to wear.

Your stratum corneum is becoming thicker as more dead skin cells linger long after their useful life. Some light exfoliation will help, as will AHA preparations (see Chapters 2 and 6). If you feel you need to turn time back, rather than just slowing it down, you might like to investigate the wrinkle-smoothing powers of some of the retinoid (vitamin-A derivative cream) preparations.

Darker patches of skin appear where abnormal melanin clumps form, but these can be lightened with topical preparations or will eventually fade if fully protected. Expression lines may now be permanently etched onto your face. Your laughter lines should be a welcome reminder of good times past, but to soften a deeply entrenched frown line, an injection of Botox or a syringe full of Hyalan gel will do the trick (see Chapters 7 and 8).

Tiny dilated, 'spider' or thread veins, may become visible as your weaker dermis is less able to hold firm the walls of the blood vessels which meander through it. These can be

will help to slow down the formation of wrinkles, 'age' spots, spider veins and also the benign solar keratoses growths which often proliferate in this decade. If it's cure rather than prevention you're after, the new generation of cosmeceuticals (see Chapter 6) can deliver impressive results, or you could opt for the more dramatic improvement given by laser treatment (see Chapter 8).

The effects of the menopause become apparent: decreased oestrogen slows the production of sebum further contributing to skin dryness. But many women find HRT or alternative remedies are a great boon to the

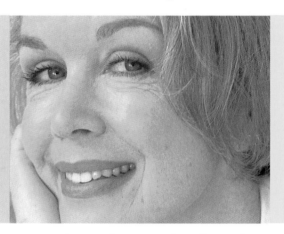

50s

60s
70s
plus

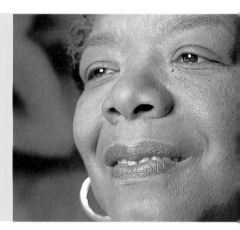

temporarily covered with make-up or permanently removed with lasers.

For as yet unknown reasons, the cells which until now produced your hair colour, cease to do so.

### In your 50s

This is the decade during which, if you haven't been using regular sunscreens, earlier sun damage really becomes apparent. If the discovery that ultraviolet rays, and not the natural ageing process, are to blame for many of the changes has come too late for you, be reassured that you can still give your skin a chance of repairing itself by using SPF15 daily. It

appearance of their skin, hair and nails as well as to their general health and wellbeing.

### In your 60s, 70s and beyond

The hormonal fluctuations which dogged your menopausal years are over and your skin enters a welcome period of relative stability. If you have regularly shielded your skin from UV rays, you will be enjoying a complexion that is smoother, brighter and less mottled than your sun-seeking counterparts. If not, and you are suffering from rucks, wrinkles, dark marks and red veins, there are many cosmetic treatments which can help you fight the ravages of time (see Chapters 7 and 9).

## The ageing process – inevitable or preventable?

**As little as 20 years ago, it was believed that the speed and degree to which your complexion crinkled was based largely on your genetic inheritance. We now know differently.**

Certain hereditary factors influence how your skin will age. You inherit your skin type (see below). You may also inherit a familial tendency to eye bags, saddle bags, a double chin or any of the other expression lines which mark out the older face from a carefree young one. Your gender, too, will affect the rate at which time takes its toll. There is, as yet, nothing you can do to change the hand you were dealt at conception. However, the appropriate skincare regime and/or a few judiciously chosen cosmetic procedures can help you to make the very best of what you were born with – and to keep it.

### The effect of skin type

The type of skin you have determines both how your skin feels and how it behaves. As you will read in Chapters 2 and 3, your skin type forms the basis for the sort of skincare regime you might wish to follow and for what sun protection you should use. It also affects, but is not solely responsible for, how your skin will stand the test of time.

Generally speaking, pale skin tends to wrinkle more rapidly than darker skin. This is largely because a darker skin tends to have more surface lipids to seal it against moisture loss, and more melanin to protect itself. On the other hand, the many wrinkles usually seen on fine, fair skin tend to be the light, crinkly variety while the thicker dermis and subcutis of the darker skin can sometimes mean its owner is more likely to develop fewer, but deeper, creases.

Wrinkles apart, other age-related changes, too, affect the different skin types: age spots, or brown spots may not be prevalent in paler skins that don't produce much melanin, but dark and numerous in an olive-skinned person who has been exposed regularly to the sun.

The thicker skin with a heavier subcutis may also be more prone to skin sag which might explain why an olive-skinned man can lose the definition of his jawline, while his Celtic wife's face, despite being traced with fine lines, remains firmly defined.

### How wrinkles form

Unlike the skin on your body which lies in sheets over the muscle, the facial skin is knitted to the musculature beneath with fingers of muscle protruding up into the dermis. This gives the face its extraordinary range of expression: it allows us to laugh, frown, scowl, smile or raise our eyebrows. How and where your face folds or creases to allow for such movements is determined both by your genes and the facial habits you develop in your lifetime. When you are young the dermis is firm and elastic enough to snap back into place and the subcutis, too, immediately smoothes down into its normal resting shape.

As you age, however, the dermis loses its spring-back capacity and the subcutaneous layer of fat ceases to return to its smooth, even state. Eventually, usually around your 40s or 50s, the puckers can no longer iron out at all and lines are indelibly etched onto your face. These changes can be kept at bay with good skincare, but a sun-weakened dermis will cease to spring back into youthful shape much earlier than a well-protected one.

### Old before your time

The genetically determined rate at which your skin ages is known as intrinsic ageing. But there

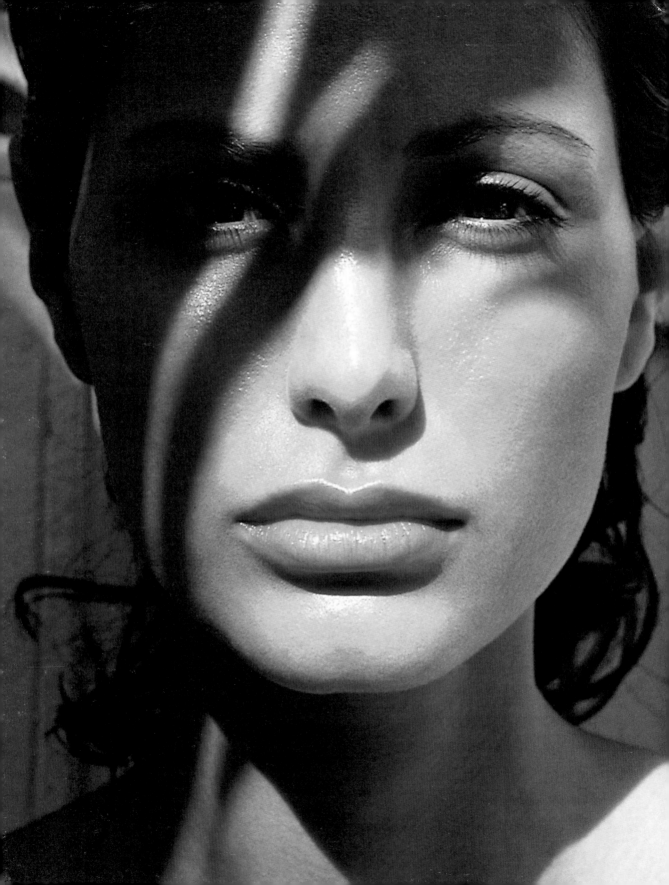

## Your Skin Type

| Type | How it looks | How it behaves |
|---|---|---|
| 1 | **Celtic**<br>Fine pored. pale to very fair, red hair, possibly freckled | High risk for skin cancers, will not tan, will freckle. Ageing risk is very high |
| 2 | **Peaches and cream**<br>Fair, fine pored | Moderately high risk for skin cancer, minimal tan, ageing and wrinkle risk high |
| 3 | **Olive**<br>Mid-European, Mediterranean, some Scandinavian | Low risk of skin cancer, high risk brown patches, wrinkle risk moderate |
| 4 | **Light Asian/Indian**<br>Hispanic, Asian, Southern Mediterranean | Very low risk of skin cancer, high risk of brown patches, wrinkle risk moderate |
| 5 | **Far Eastern**<br>Some Asian-Indian, Polynesian | Very low risk of skin cancer, pigment of brown patches high, wrinkle risk low |
| 6 | **Light black**<br>African, African-American, West Indian | Very low risk of skin cancer, pigment of brown patches high, wrinkle risk low |
| 7 | **Deep black**<br>Central African, some Afro-Caribbean, Australian Aborigine | Extremely low risk of skin cancer, resisitant to sun damage, wrinkle risk low |

*Great skin such as this is dependent on more than youth and good genes – happily much of it within our control.*

is a far more powerful force in the ageing equation: the sun. There are few among us who don't grumble about getting old, too soon. In terms of your skin, the complaint is very valid because the sun's rays do indeed age your skin faster than time alone can. Its ultraviolet and infrared rays irradiate bits of DNA and cause thermal injury. The destruction itself and the concentration of effort required to repair it, speeds up the natural ageing process many times over. Skin which is sun-damaged beyond its years is referred to as prematurely-aged or photo-damaged.

In fact, some dermatologists go far as to say that up to 80 per cent of ageing signs are due to photo-damage while others, myself included, are reluctant to put such a figure on it. There is no absolutely no doubt that the sun prematurely ages the skin, but I feel that we do not yet know enough to specifically quantify the extent of that acceleration.

### The dangerous rays

The sun emits rays of varying wavelengths. Physicists divide its ultraviolet rays into A – the longer, more lethargic length, B – which are shorter and more energetic, and C – which are so frenetic that it has the power to mutate the DNA of all living things. (Happily, the ozone layer still filters out almost all UVC since if much of it got through it would actually threaten life on earth.)

Both UVA and UVB reach the earth's surface and are a menace to our skin. UVB is often called the 'burning' ray as it is primarily responsible for the visible and sometimes very painful effects of sunburn. It also dries out your skin and most importantly increases your risk of skin cancer.

UVA is often known as the 'ageing' ray because it generally causes the wrinkling and sagging that, as little as 15 years ago, were thought of as the natural, and inevitable part of the ageing process.

### Free radicals – ageing menace to your skin

They may sound like the scaremongering pseudo-scientific invention of a cosmetics' marketeer but free radicals are a real, destructive force in the everyday life of every cell of your body. A free radical, also known as a radical oxide, is a rogue molecule created during the natural cell oxidation process. Devoid of a crucial electron, it will endeavour to wrest one from wherever it can, often tearing apart healthy body cells in the process. When it does so, it creates more electron-missing molecules and so a vicious circle of damage begins. A certain number of free radicals in the body is perfectly normal. Indeed, some help to combat bacteria, fight malignant cells, and can dilate blood vessels and affect blood clotting. But many are highly destructive and can irreversibly damage nucleic acids, proteins, lipids and the skin's connective tissues.

Our bodies are well equipped to fight off these vicious molecules with natural antioxidants such as superoxide dismutase, glutathione and melanin. It can also get help from vitamins A, C and E which give up their electrons for the greater good of our cells. But when the number of free radicals overwhelms the available electrons, healthy cells are the victims. Free radical damage makes the cells more vulnerable to degenerative diseases, not just of our skin, but of all body tissues. Much of today's disease and anti-ageing research is now focused on the preventive effects of a diet rich in antioxidant vitamins.

Under the sun, or in a toxic environment radical production in the skin is vastly accelerated. It is estimated, however, that as little as 1 per cent of the vitamins that we take in make it through to our skin and for this reason dermatologists and cosmetic scientists are attempting to boost our skin's free radical scavenging power by applying antioxidant vitamins directly to the skin.

In fact, in France, a recently completed satellite study of the government sponsored Supplementation Vitamin and Mineral Antioxidant trial revealed that antioxidant vitamins applied to the skin help to defend the skin against free radical damage. The results showed that vitamins applied to the skin gave it such efficient protection, that it was able to go about its natural repair process unchallenged by further assault. The net result is that not only does skin not deteriorate, but it actually improves as damage already done is, to a degree, undone. (For more on free radicals and antioxidant skin creams, see Chapters 2 and 3.)

**beauty spot**

Unlike natural ageing, over which you are powerless, premature ageing is preventable. And if you consider that premature ageing may account for up to 80 per cent of the marks and lines that define the older face that's a lot of age you can save.

*To tan or not to tan? There is no question that doing all you can to shield your skin from the sun's ageing ray is your best bet for great looking skin, now and forever.*

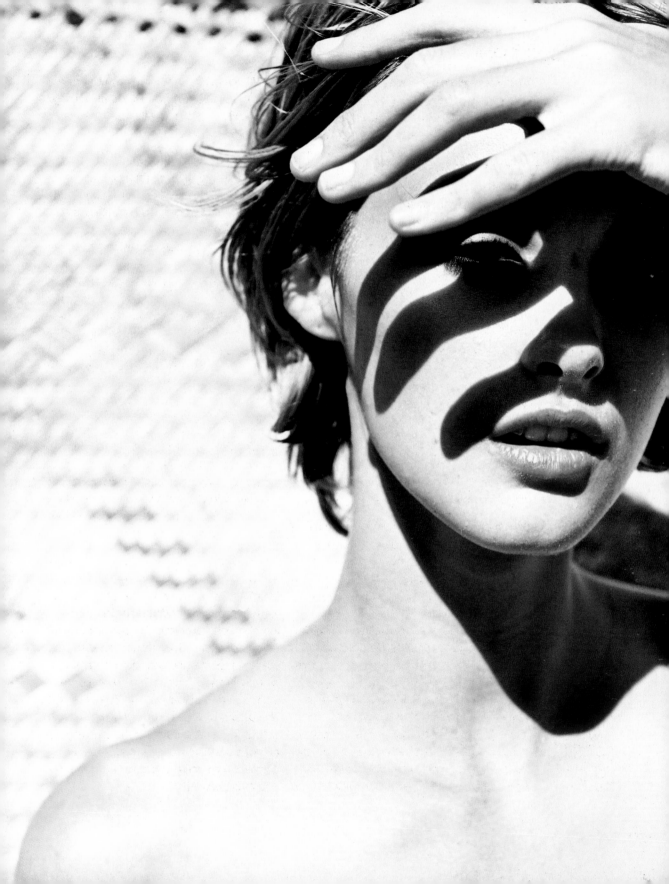

## Other factors in the ageing process

**It is not only the sun that prematurely ages the skin. Anything that disrupts your skin's optimum daily routine, pollutes it, or generates excessive free radical activity will also speed up its rate of decline.**

### Toxins and other triggers

**Cigarette smoke** The effects are threefold. Firstly, smoking constricts the capillaries restricting blood flow to the tiny vessels of the dermis. This means less oxygen and fewer nutrients are carried in, while waste products are not as efficiently carried away, the net result of which is compromised skin function. Secondly, the repeated action of pursing the lips to draw on the cigarette causes the more rapid formation of lines. Thirdly, cigarette smoke is a potent source of free radicals. And you don't even need to smoke the cigarette yourself to suffer this effect, just being in a smoky room induces a marked increase in free radical activity in the skin.

> If you are a smoker you can fortify your skin's free radical quenching capability with antioxidant face creams

If you are a smoker and can't give up, you can fortify your skin's free radical quenching capacity with antioxidant face creams and your entire body's defence mechanisms with a diet rich in vitamins A, C and E.

**Pollution** The airborne toxins in urban and industrial environments have a similar action to cigarette smoke. They deprive you and your skin of oxygen and generate free radicals. Despite the absence of much hard clinical data, it is now considered a worthwhile safeguard to wear daily sunscreens supplemented with antioxidant vitamins to help offset the effects of pollution.

Almost all skincare ranges, from dermatologists' own to mass-market, now contain sophisticated cocktails of the best known free radical scavengers (see Chapter 2).

**Inflammation** Just as it is now known that stressed personalities age faster than their care-free counterparts, skin that is under stress will tend to age more rapidly. Whether the redness you see is because of sunburn, physically injury, something you applied to it, or even eczema, the effect is the same. Free radicals are produced, they go on the rampage, and instead of going about its daily maintenance schedule, your skin has to stop and do some major repairs. This is important to remember when buying and applying skin creams; if your face flares up in protest when you apply with the latest anti-ageing potion, it is likely that it is having the very opposite effect of the one you were hoping for.

### The effects of food and drink

**Alcohol** If you drink more than moderate amounts on a very regular basis the constant dilating of the facial blood vessels that alcohol induces puts a lot of pressure on the collagen and elastin of the dermis which support the walls of those blood vessels. However, if you are young and you don't sunbathe, your dermis could probably cope for a good while but as you get older and collagen and elastin are damaged by UV exposure, they will no longer contain the walls of the blood vessels and small dilated capillaries show up on your face as thread veins. Alcohol also robs your skin of vitamins and minerals, and for this reason it is often known as an anti-nutrient.

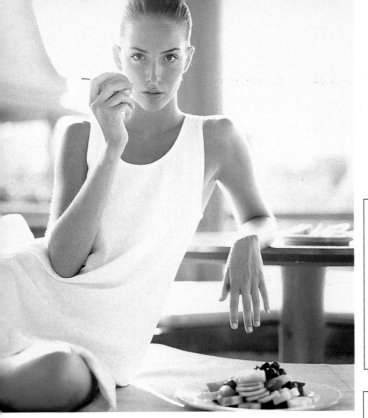

*Eating plenty of fresh fruit and vegetables containing antioxidant vitamins such as A, beta carotene, B and C may help prevent some of the free radical damage which contributes to premature skin ageing. And to supplement what can't get through to your skin from the inside, many skin products now contain similar sorts of antioxidant vitamins.*

various vitamins and minerals. Taking massive doses of say, vitamin C, without enough of its co-factors, such as zinc, is at best wasteful. In the case of vitamin A, high doses can actually be toxic (high levels of vitamin A can cause liver damage).

**Vitamin C** This is one of the most important vitamins in the manufacture of strong, healthy skin. It is used by the dermis to manufacture collagen. An extreme lack of this particular vitamin causes scurvy, the well-known disease that affected the skin and gums of ancient sea-farers. But it is possible that diets even slightly deficient in vitamin C might compromise the production of collagen.

**Vitamin E** Although there is no known deficiency disease associated with this vitamin, it is now being hailed as a 'radical protector'. Vitamin E is known to work well with the more unstable C molecule, re-fortifying it to fight on against free radicals.

**Thiamine** This is one of the B vitamins, and it is known to be important in ensuring normal cellular exchanges in skin, hair and nails.

**Zinc** is essential for normal epidermal cell growth.

**Selenium** is an essential element in the production of glutathione, our natural free-radical scavenger.

**Calcium** is a key mineral to helping epidermal cells mature.

## Diet

Despite the number of supplements available at chemists and supermarkets promising to bestow beautiful skin upon you, mainstream nutritionists still insist that it is possible to get all we need from a well-balanced diet. However, your skin may be the last organ to benefit from the nutrients you ingest. It is thought that as little as 1% of vitamins and trace elements become available to it, hence the great attention being focused on topical applications (see Chapter 2).

Below is a list of the most important vitamins and minerals in the growth and maintenance of healthy skin, hair and nails. But be aware that if you suspect that, despite an ample pair of hips, or because of a bony pair, your diet may be lacking, the best way to supplement it is by taking a well-formulated multi-vitamin and mineral capsule. Your skin, like all the organs of your body, requires a fine balance of all the

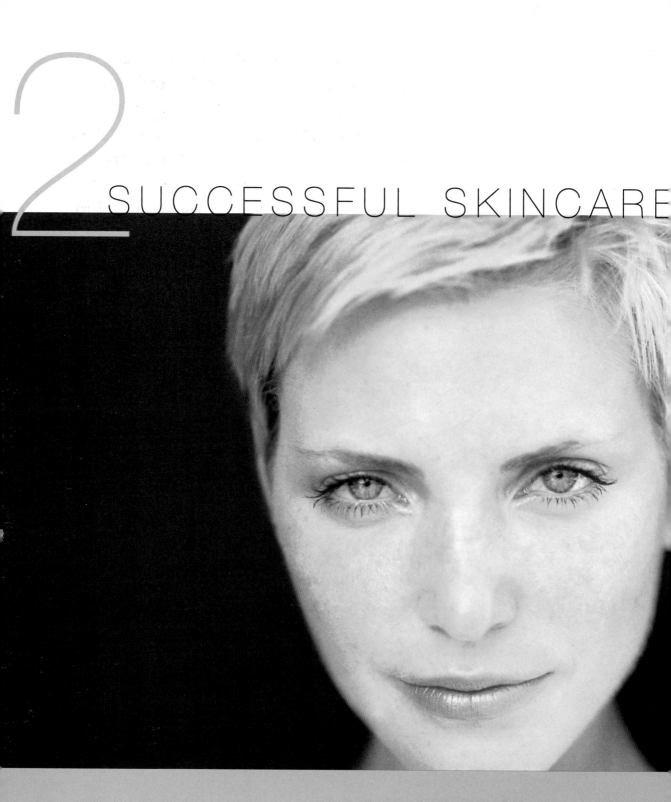

# 2 SUCCESSFUL SKINCARE

**Are you confused about what you should or should not be putting on your face? Seductive marketing, coupled with a lack of good scientific data, makes it difficult for even the beauty literate to develop a clear idea of how best to care for her skin.**

# the skincare

question we are both most keenly, asked – by both seasoned skin cream aficionados and ardent sceptics alike, is 'what should I be using?' Unfortunately, as you probably suspected, there is no straightforward answer. Good skincare is less a matter of what you use than what you do. And what you do depends on your own particular skin and how it behaves.

When it comes to a skincare regime, everyone tends to think of the beauty consultant's mantra of 'cleanse, tone, and moisturize'. However, science supports the need for just two: cleanse and, only if necessary, moisturize. The dermatologists' basics of good facial skincare are more action-than product-based.

They are as follows:

1   Correctly determine your skin type.

2   Keep your face scrupulously clean.

3   Keep your skin adequately moisturized.

4   Protect your skin from the sun.

## What is my skin type?

Many of you will already instinctively know what type of skin you have, or you will have been told by a beauty professional in the department store or salon. However, if you do get it wrong, or are wrongly advised, your skin can suffer – so too, can your pocket as you waste money on products that hinder rather than help.

## Combination skin

If your complexion has some oily areas, such as the T-zone that runs across your forehead, down your nose and chin, but others areas of your face such as your cheeks and neck are normal to dry, you have this type of skin. About 40 per cent of women have combination skin.

## Oily skin

If your skin usually feels greasy, is often shiny, can be prone to spots and has visible, open pores, you have this skin type.

## Dry skin

If your skin often feels tight and stretched, particularly after washing; if you never have greasy feeling areas, if you have flaky patches of skin or if you are very fair skinned, you probably have this skin type.

## Normal skin

If your skin is neither particularly greasy, nor dry, you probably have this type of skin. If you don't know if it's greasy or dry, its probably normal. It might sound rather dull, but just be thankful.

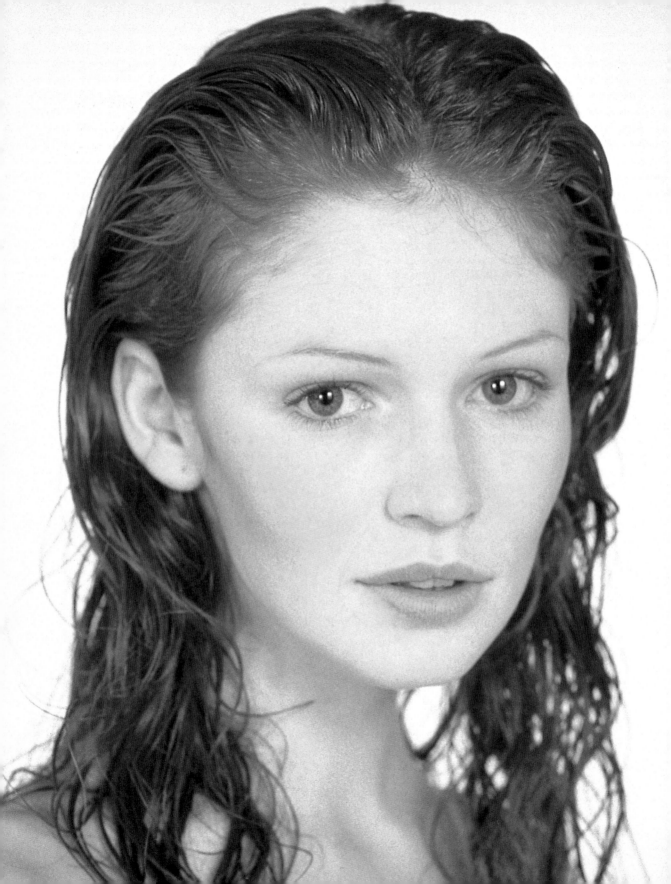

# Cleansing

**If you want your skin to look and feel good, careful cleansing is important. But how do you choose the right cleanser for you from the many different types of cosmetic cleanser stacked on shelves in every cosmetics hall, supermarket and chemist? There are tissue-off cleansing milks, wash-off gels, AHA rinse-away liqui-gels and soap-free soap bars. The choice can be paralysing but getting the right one is the cornerstone of successful skincare.**

It's easy to think of cleansing as a necessary evil, the boring precursor to the really exciting business of applying your moisturizing, cellular regenerating, anti-ageing serum. In many respects, however, cleansing is one of the most important steps in your skincare regime. If you experience spots, dry or sensitive skin, it is worth looking closely at your cleansing regime. If you aren't washing thoroughly enough, dirt can clog pores and cause spots. On the other hand, if you are constantly stripping away essential skin oils which your skin isn't capable of replacing you will dry out your stratum corneum and make your skin less able hold its own moisture (which after all, is better for it than anything you can buy). If your chosen cleanser is wrong for your skin, it won't matter what anti-spot treatments, moisturizers or skin calmers you use because the root of your skin-ills will lie elsewhere.

## The soap and water debate

For many skins, there's little wrong with soap and water face washing. However, this is provided you don't normally wear make-up, you have normal to oily skin, and you live in an area where the water is normal to soft. Otherwise, you will find three main problems with soap.

Soap isn't very good at removing make-up, because unlike cosmetic cleansers it does not have enough oils to dissolve make-up, which cosmetic scientists have created to have great staying power.

*If your skin is fair and frail, the first step to successful skincare lies in extremely gentle cleansing.*

Soap can be very drying on the skin as it can dissolve and wash away skin oils and/or lipids which act as a sealant to the stratum corneum. Normal skin should be able to make up this lipid deficiency within a few hours, but a dry skin often won't generate enough lipids to make up the shortfall within 24 hours – that is, before you next wash your face.

Skin is naturally acidic with a pH balance of around 5.5, but soap is generally alkaline or pH 8 or higher. If you use alkaline soap with hard water you will find that it's hard to rinse off or you will get some scum residue. If some of this remains on your skin, it can upset its natural acid balance and may continue to 'dissolve' skin lipids long after the washing process is over.

### Choosing your cosmetic cleanser

Cosmetic cleansers are carefully formulated to dissolve the most tenacious of make-up formulations, excess skin oils and dirt. The very best cleanser is one that quickly and efficiently does so and rinses cleanly away. It is also one which leaves enough skin lipids in place so that you skin is comfortably supple but not so many that your pores are clogged with them. It's a fine balancing act that can mean the difference between dry, spotty or fabulously clear skin. The formulating chemist will have spent weeks in the laboratory making sure that his or her product fills the above criteria. You will have to rely on yourself, or a sales consultant to ensure you're getting the one that is right for your skin.

In the past, those with dry skin were ordered to use cleansing milks or lotions while oilier types were prescribed foaming washes or non-soap bar cleansers. Today, there are no such hard and fast rules, not least because cosmetics companies are now reluctant to be patronizingly dictatorial towards their increasingly knowledgeable customers. But how, then, to choose between the myriad of pink gel washes and creamy cleansing lotions available?

As long as the product cleanses efficiently, your skin is clear and comfortable afterwards and you like using it, you've got the right product. The only stipulation we have is to look for formulations that wash away with water. The rinsing action is extremely gentle – tissuing can be harsh on frail skins and may not remove enough to keep oily skins spot free. The water will also help to soothe and hydrate the skin.

## Soap or cleansers – the pros and cons

| Type of cleanser | + plus | - minus |
| --- | --- | --- |
| **Household soap** | Efficient cleanser | Tends to leave alkaline residue if used in hard water. Can be excessively drying to all but very oily skins. |
| **Superfatted soap** | Contains more fatty substances such as moisturizing cream, lanolin and cocoa butter so is less drying. | Less efficient cleansing because the fatty residue left on the skin probably also contains some dirt – it's very difficult for a soap to do the two very different jobs of washing and moisturizing. |
| **Transparent or glycerine soap** | Contains more fats and glycerin, known for its humectant, or water-attracting properties. | Lathers less well and is used up more quickly than regular soap. It is more expensive to make and therefore to buy. |
| **Liquid or gel cleansers** | Contains detergents made from petroleum products. Detergent often frightens off skincare consumers because it makes them think of their dishwashing liquid, but the synthetic detergents in liquid cleansers are developed specifically for gentle facial cleansing. The detergents do not interact with hard water salts so soap scum residue isn't a problem. | If you are concerned about the effects of the petroleum industry on the environment, you may prefer to use a more 'natural' soap product. |
| **Non-soap bar cleanser** | This is the solid version of the above, and is often aimed at oilier skins. It may contain more detergents, and cleanses more efficiently. | More expensive than traditional soap and may be drying to sensitive skins. |
| **Cleansing milks or lotions** | Essentially oil and water emulsions. The oil picks up the make-up so that it can be wiped or rinsed away. These formulations for dry skins limit the oil which is removed from the skin. | May not remove enough sebum to keep oily skin clean and prevent spots. |
| **Cleansing Oils** | Normally vegetable oils with some emulsifiers so that they rinse well with water. Good for dry skins; rapidly melts make-up. | May not remove enough oil, or indeed may contribute too much oil to greasy skins. |

# Toning

**Not long ago the accepted skincare routine was: cleanse – tone – moisturize. However, with the advent of rinse-off cleansers, separate toners are becoming less necessary.**

When greasy cold creams and milky cleansers were standard make-up removers a separate toning lotion was always used to remove any oily residue. But the modern, rinse-off cleansers rarely require the services of a toner.

The word 'toner' is, of course, a bit of a misnomer; we can't expect a mixture of water, alcohol, and/or astringent or emollient agents to permanently firm or recondition our skin. Toners are formulated to remove the oily cleanser residue or natural skin sebum, or simply to impart a feeling of freshness. 'Degreaser', however, isn't a particularly seductive word and a 'refresher' isn't something consumers are likely to want to hand over much money for.

Toners may no longer be essential, but they do have their uses. If you like using a milky cleanser, for instance, or one that doesn't rinse well, you will need to dissolve and wipe away residual dirt and grease. If your skin is oily and you want to quickly cleanse and refresh it before going out in the evening, for example, applying some toner will be very effective. They can also act as a more fragrant alternative to a splash of cold tap water in the morning.

## Types of toner

There are two types of toner, the first for oily skin, which is essentially a solvent and is used after milky or oil cleansers. It may contain up to 70 per cent alcohol and/or exfoliating salicylic acid, astringents such as witch hazel, or solvents such as resorcinol, along with colours and fragrance. The second variety of toner is formulated for normal or dry skin and contains little or no alcohol or other solvents but has emollient compounds such as allantoin or glycerine, soothing plant extracts and pleasant scents instead.

Much is often claimed for toners, little of it possible. When they are used for oily skin they will certainly remove grease, but can't stop your skin producing it. And while they might appear to shrink your pores, in reality the solvent has probably simply temporarily irritated your skin sufficiently to inflame the tissue around the pore. Toners for dry skin might also leave your face feeling less stretched and taut than after washing alone, but they can't put sufficient moisture back into the skin for any long-term therapeutic effect.

Just as over-cleansing can strip away the oils your skin needs to keep it healthy, so can excessive use of the wrong toner. If your skin is very greasy, it will probably happily tolerate the use of a 70 per cent alcohol-based, salicylic acid containing toner. If it's dry, however, the solvents could dissolve essential lipids causing the skin to become dehydrated. So use toners cautiously and be guided by the reaction of your skin.

### beauty spot

**The received wisdom that, with age, men get better while women do not, does, infuriatingly, has some basis in medical fact. Men have more of the sex hormone androgen giving them a thicker dermis and subcutis which stands them in useful stead for later life.**

## Moisturizing

**For those with dry skin, the moisturizer is an essential staple – a source of soothing and protective hydration. For others, its application may be an unnecessary step in their skincare regime. But deciding if or when to moisturize is only half the problem; there is a bewildering array of products from which to choose.**

Moisturizers divide into oil-in-water or water-in-oil (or sometimes even water-in-oil-in-water) emulsions. In the former, the microdroplets of oil are held within the water so that the cream feels lighter and often slicker, while in the latter the water is held within the oil making the preparations slightly richer feeling. The water hydrates the skin while the oil helps to seal in the water.

Day creams tend to be based on the light oil-in-water emulsions while night creams, which don't have to go under make-up, are the heavier water-in-oil variety. Modern cosmetic technology, however, has recently developed the oil-free moisturizer where the oils that act as softeners and moisture sealants are replaced by a light oil-mimicking substance such as silicone. These creams are a welcome advance particularly for normal, combination or oily skins as some oils can clog up the skin. Very dry skins which are deficient in both oils and water, however, may still benefit from the more traditional oil and water emulsions.

### beauty spot

**The outer layer of healthy skin is about 10 per cent water. Oddly, there is precious little difference between the water levels of oily and dry skin. Rather, dry skin is deficient in the fatty lipids which help seal skin against moisture loss. Dry skins, therefore, benefit from moisturizers rich in natural lipid-mimicking ingredients.**

Beyond the basic water and oil components, formulators add a variety of substances to help remedy the cause and symptoms of dry skin: humectants like glycerin and hyaluronic acid which attract water from your environment and hold it on your skin; ceramides which help seal the cells of the stratum corneum together; and essential fatty acids such as linoleic acid and vitamin F to help rebuild the lipids layers which may be deficient in dry skins.

### When to moisturize

One of the key things to remember is that not everyone needs to moisturize – at least not all the time, or indeed all over. As a general rule, if ten minutes after washing your face with a gentle cleanser your face still feels taut and tight you probably need to apply a moisturizer. But if you have oily skin and it only ever feels taut and tight occasionally, just moisturize occasionally to suit. Many women find their skin needs moisturizer during the low-humidity winter months, but does not need it during the summer months. This is quite normal. Just be guided by how your skin feels and behaves.

Given the amount of skincare advice on offer from eager beauty sales staff in department stores, it is very easy to fall into the trap of thinking that they know best. They know a lot, particularly about the products they make and sell, but what they can't know is how your skin feels or how it reacts during the day and night. The key to successful skincare lies in learning to understand what your skin is telling you.

If and when you decide your face needs a moisturizer, (and, from their 20s on, approximately 50 per cent of women do), the seemingly unlimited choice can cause more problems. You should use a good quality moisturizer that makes your skin feel comfortable without overloading it. Modern cosmetic science is now highly sophisticated and you would be hard-pressed to find a badly formulated cream on the market.

When buying a moisturizer, decide for yourself what you're looking for and then listen to what the consultant has to say, or what the accompanying information offers, only in as much as it helps you to determine whether it's what you need. Again, make full use of samples and trial sizes.

sunscreens and, possibly, with antioxidant back up (see antioxidants page 38). At night, obviously, sun protection is redundant but replenishing any moisture lost during the day and feeding in active agents useful in optimum skin function becomes important.

As you have read, not long ago it was believed that nothing could really penetrate the skin but it is now known that much can. It has also recently become clear that the process of absorption is best at night. Studies show that transepidermal water-loss, more

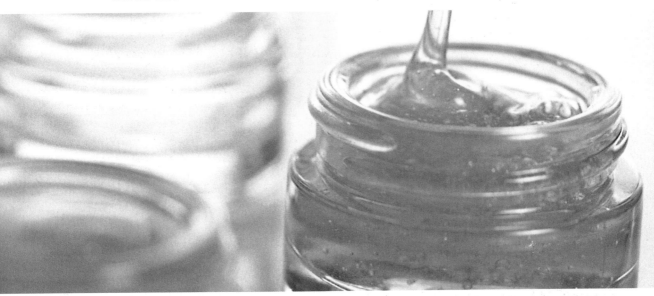

The best time to use a moisturizer is at night. During the day it is preferable to use a day cream with sunscreens, which although it will probably contain moisturizing ingredients will mainly protect your skin.

### Night and day preparations – what's the difference?

It is tempting to think that different creams exist only to persuade us to buy two where one would do. In most cases, however, it is sensible to have separate day and night creams. During the day, your skin requires protection from the elements, so you will want to apply a cream with

conveniently known as TEWL, is greatest at night – you may have read the fascinating figures of how much sweat our mattresses soak up as we sleep. And, as water leaches out of the skin, so other things gain entry.

Whatever your skin type, therefore, whether you're concerned about feeding back in moisture, or benefiting from cosmeceuticals such as tretinoin, AHAs or ascorbic acid (see Chapter 6), the basis of any successful skincare regime is to protect during the day and to 'treat' the skin at night. Prevention is followed by, we hope, a degree of cure.

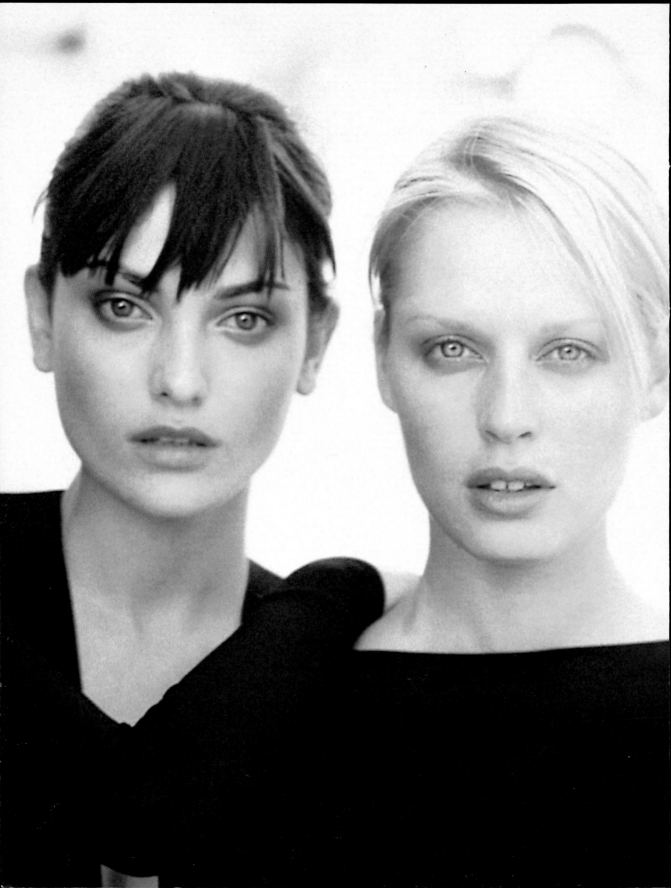

## Good daily facial skincare regimes

| Skin type | morning | night |
|---|---|---|
| **dry** | 1 Splash face with water or gently and lightly stroke with a cotton wool pad soaked with non-alcohol based toner. 2 Pat dry. 3 Apply moisturizing daily sunscreen (minimum SPF15-20) to face and neck. | 1 Wash face with rinse-off, non-soap cleanser (milk or gel). 2 Pat dry. 3 If using AHA or retinoid, apply now. Wait ten minutes for active preparations to penetrate. Apply moisturizing/nourishing night cream to face. |
| **normal** | 1 Wash face with non-soap cleanser. 2 Pat dry. 3 Apply moisturizing daily sunscreen (min SPF15-20) to face and neck. | 1 Wash face with rinse-off, non-soap cleanser (milk or gel). 2 Pat dry. 3 If using AHA or retinoid, apply now. Wait ten minutes. If skin still feels dry, apply moisturizing/nourishing night cream. |
| **combination** | 1 Wash T-zone only with non-soap cleanser or remove nose, chin or forehead grease with a toner-soaked cotton pad (one with a low alcohol content is fine). 2 Pat dry. 3 Apply oil-free daily sunscreen (minimum SPF 15–20) and if needed, a richer moisturizer to any dry areas. | 1 Wash with rinse-off, non-soap cleanser (gel rather than milk). 2 Pat dry. 3 If using AHA or retinoid, apply now. Wait ten minutes for active preparations to penetrate. 4 Apply moisturizing/nourishing night cream, if necessary, to dry areas such as cheeks and around the eyes. |
| **oily** | 1 Wash face with oily skin specific non-soap cleanser. 2 Pat dry. 3 Apply oil-free daily sunscreen (minimum SPF15–20) to face and neck. | 1 Wash face with soap or oily skin specific non-soap cleanser 2 If necessary, use alcohol-based toner. 3 Apply AHA or retinoid preparation. (Moisturizer is probably not required, except perhaps over cheeks and neck). |

*Whether your skintype is Mediterranean or Nordic, the basic principles of skincare are the same. The difference lies in the details.*

## Beyond the basics

**Cleansing, moisturizing and sunscreening may be the keystones of good skincare but department store and pharmacy shelves are festooned with many other skincare products: masks, exfoliators, intensive serums... Do such products fit into the scientifically sound skincare regime? And if so, where?**

### Masks

Your skin won't suddenly shrivel up or break out in spots if you don't use a mask on the weekly basis the cosmetics companies usually suggest. But that doesn't mean they're not of benefit, and not just psychologically as you take time out to apply one. A very oily skin may well be cleared of greasy debris with a cleansing clay mask, a fraught skin might be soothed by a cool gel mask and a dry skin might feel more supple and look more radiant after a moisturizing mask.

Yet again, be guided by your skin, not by marketing blurb or sales pitches. If you're using a heavy-duty moisturizer and still have dry skin, you might like to try a hydrating mask twice a week. If your oily skins persists in developing spots, try a clay-based mask up to three times a week. If your problem-free skin ain't broke...

**beauty spot**

**Make-up nowadays has similar skincare ingredients to those found in specialist skin creams. Foundations and lipsticks, in particular, contains ingredients such as humectants, antioxidant vitamins, sun blockers and ceramides, which can be every bit as useful in your daily skincare regime as skin creams.**

### Exfoliators

Exfoliating is another one of those tasks the skincare companies advise you to do at least once of week. But is there any medical basis for the practice? Yes. Essentially, exfoliating involves the removal of dead skin cells and debris. In both oily and dry skins exfoliation can be a useful aid in the prevention of the most common problems of each type – spots in oily skin, and a dull, flaky skin appearance in dry.

In the past, exfoliating was done quite simply by rubbing off the dead cells, either with a face cloth, with the softer, facial equivalent of the pot scourer, or with a special cosmetic scrub containing abrasive particles such as ground walnut kernel or, more recently, smooth spherical synthetic particles. All of these were physical exfoliators.

Today there are new creams which will remove dead skin cells without recourse to rubbing. Alpha hydroxy acids, chemicals found naturally in, amongst other things, sugar cane, apples, soured milk and pawpaw (see page 37) are incorporated into leave-on face creams. The acid content dissolves the protein bond which keeps a dead skin cell hanging on beyond its useful life, thereby smoothing and clarifying the complexion. As long as the cream doesn't contain an acid concentration of any more than about 10 per cent, there's little chance of removing more cells that you can comfortably afford to lose. Most dermatologists now prefer to recommend the use of AHAs over physical sloughing agents largely because the dose is carefully controlled and there is less chance of physical injury.

Overdo exfoliation, however, and things can go wrong. It doesn't take a mathematician to work out that with a cell turnover rate of 28 days, you can't force off five layers of the total twenty-odd keratinocytes that make up the stratum corneum

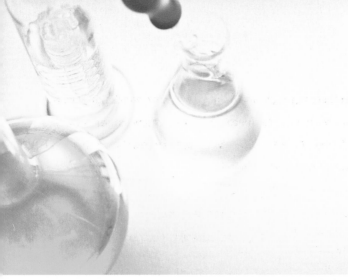

### Eye on eye creams

The worried possessor of a rapidly developing pair of crow's feet is easy prey for the cosmetics hounds. However, using a specialist eye cream can help. Oil glands in the eye area are less active than those in the T-zone and the skin is much thinner than elsewhere on your face so it tends to be more easily irritated. Eye creams are therefore usually formulated with potent moisturizers but fewer potentially irritating active ingredients.

*Without independent clinical trials, it's hard to know what value there may be in the sorts of intensive serums offered within many cosmetics ranges, above. The very fine skin around the eye, right, presents a particular challenge to cosmetic scientists – creams must fight wrinkles without being irritating.*

without going into the red – which is exactly the shade your face will be if you overdo it. You won't just rid your face of its dead skin, but of its defensive barrier to the outside world. And that is something your skin finds deeply irritating. If you want a more radical skin smoothing effect, the physicians version of exfoliation is the peel. For details see Chapter 8.

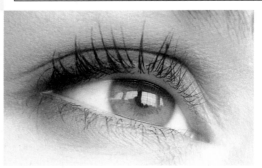

### Serums

Generally, serums tend not to be particularly moisturizing but are formulated with what the men in white coats at the cosmetic labs believe to be an extra special skin energizing ingredient – a vitamin, perhaps, or an enzyme, an amino acid or an anti-flammatory agent. Each company will have its own clinical data to support the benefits of their own given product but with no independent investigation into the merits of any such formulations you will have to make your own decision as to whether you think your skin could benefit from such a product.

### The sum of the parts

There are face creams and eye gels, lip salves and neck firmers, bust gels and thigh toners. It's very easy to take the cynic's view and say that skincare companies are cravenly creating a need for as many different creams as they think

the market will tolerate. However, there is a case to be argued for different formulations for different body parts not least because our skincare concern differs with each area. Most women want soft, full lips but taut, firm thighs; gleaming shoulders but matt noses; they want to firm up their jawlines but soften the lines around their eyes.

Many of the decisions you make about the cosmetic preparations you buy are probably partly based on how attractive the product feels to you. This is the right way to consider all areas of your body. Of course, skin is skin. Whether it's thick, rough foot skin or thin, delicate eye skin, its needs are similar: protection from the sun, gentle cleansing and sufficient moisture. What varies is the degree of protection or moisture each area requires: shins need more moisture; hands need more sun protection.

# Chapter Two

## Sensitive skin

**In Britain, 80 per cent of women say they suffer from sensitive skin. The latest understanding of what makes some skins so intolerant of all our best efforts to help it involves the most superficial skin layer – the stratum corneum.**

Until recently, the sensitive-skinned used to receive little sympathy from physicians because their mild- to irritatingly-persistent burning, itching or prickling sensations often exhibited no visible symptoms. However, new diagnostic tools, such as Doppler ultrasound, have shown what is causing their problem. The device, which traces blood flow, revealed that when sensitive skin prickles, there is indeed increased blood flow. Further investigation also showed traces of the body's inflammatory protein, histamine, in irritated areas. This sort of sensitivity reaction was dubbed 'sub clinical irritation' and the proof of its existence lead physicians to seek the cause. The vast majority of women who claim to have sensitive skin are those with dry skin and so the stratum corneum came under scrutiny.

In women with sensitive skin, it became apparent that the stratum corneum's barrier function was often seriously compromised. Deficient in lipids, the stratum corneum was allowing excessive water loss, so the skin was perpetually 'drying out', and potential irritants were allowed in. Modern cosmetic dermatologists now believe that sensitive skin is less 'born that way' than 'made' – that while we might inherit an irritation-prone skin, it's actually what we do to it on a daily basis that breaks down its defences and lowers its tolerance levels.

### Special care for fragile skin

In caring for sensitive skin the aim is threefold. Firstly, to ensure you don't further compromise your skin's barrier function, secondly, to build up its outer defences and thirdly to use, or do to it, nothing that gives it cause to get upset. Buy only skincare ranges that are made for sensitive skin. They are free of many of the ingredients that can irritate. Wash your face in the evening only, using very gentle cleanser that you feel still washes your face efficiently. Protect your skin from UV rays to help prevent any damage to the lipids of your stratum corneum. If you have problems using a sunscreen try one containing physical sun blockers as opposed to chemical-based ones. (Look for zinc oxide or titanium dioxide in the ingredients listed.)

Don't use toners or alcohol-based astringents. If you can't resist using a toner, choose an alcohol-free hydrating one.

Remove flaky skin with a mild AHA product rather than a scouring pad. (AHAs can also help to improve your skin's moisture-holding ability.) But don't use any products that sting, burn or make your skin itch.

### beauty spot

**Cosmetic ranges for sensitive skin are usually marked hypoallergenic and are formulated without ingredients that are well-known to cause either allergic or more mild skin reactions. However hypoallergenic doesn't mean that you can't react to it, simply that you are less likely to.**

## What's in a cream?

**Nowadays when you buy a skin cream the number of ingredients it contains can be baffling: AHAs, liposomes, ceramides, collagen, NMF – the list is endless. Having a basic understanding of what they can do to your skin will help you to choose the product you want.**

### Common ingredients

#### Ceramides

The body makes a variety of ceramides, several of which are found in the skin. Ceramides help to keep the skin cells functioning well. Dry skin is often deficient in ceramides so some skin cream manufacturers synthesize them to help back up the skin's natural defences. It's unclear whether topically applied ceramides can do the job of the natural variety, but they probably temporarily help to improve barrier function.

#### Liposomes

*Citric acid is one of a number of alpha hydroxy, or fruit acids, currently in cosmetic use for its skin smoothing properties.*

These were developed for pharmaceutical purposes to carry drugs into our systems via the skin rather than the gut. They are hollow spheres made up of lipids similar to the skin's own so are readily accepted by the skin. Quickly commandeered for cosmetic use, they are now pumped full of active skin ingredients in the hope they will carry them into to the deeper layers of the epidermis. Early liposomes were relatively big and deposited large amounts of active ingredient soon after application. The newer generation are smaller in the hope that they can penetrate further and release smaller amounts of active ingredient over greater periods of time. Each company has its own name for them, such as 'nanospheres' and 'micelles'.

#### AHAs – Alpha hydroxy acids

These are also known as fruit acids because some are found in citrus fruits (citric), apples (malic) and papaya (pyruvic) and because, from a marketing point of view, 'fruit' sounds like a comfortingly natural thing to be putting on your face. Other acids in the family include lactic acid (from milk), tartaric acid (from red wine), and the most exciting and therefore most widely researched, glycolic acid (from sugar cane).

Lactic acid has been used to soften skin for centuries and resurfaced in modern cosmetic creams in the 70s after studies showed that combined with sodium lactate, it improved the skin's moisture-holding capacity. Tartaric acid, too, has been in used for years: French women used to apply red wine to their faces. Collectively, AHAs have recently been in the vanguard of the new cosmeceutical movement as they are used to formulate creams which perform beyond the normally superficial cosmetic role.

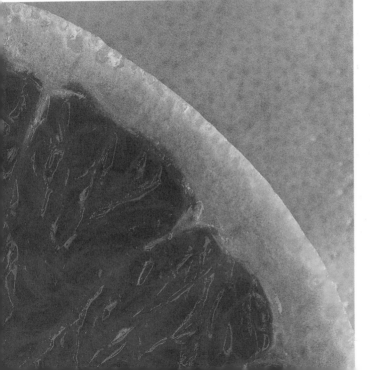

In the late 80s Dr Eugene van Scott and his partner Dr Ruey Yu reported that the dead skin cells build-up which gave icthyosis sufferers their crocodile-skin appearance could be alleviated with an glycolic acid preparation.

They showed that the acid molecule dissolved the protein bond which kept a dead skin cell attached. Not only did glycolic acid prove capable of normalizing the desquamation process but could also improve the skin's own moisture-retaining capability.

Dermatologists use AHAs in concentrations up to 70 per cent to perform acid peels and prescribe 5–20 per cent AHA creams (see Chapters 7 and 9). The percentage contained in cosmetic creams varies from 1–7 per cent. Some over-the-counter pharmacy brands contain between 5–15 per cent.

Cosmetic AHA preparations can help keep the skin free of dulling and skin-pore-clogging dead cells. They can make the skin slightly brighter and improve its moisture retention. Unlike the physician-prescribed higher concentrations, they cannot produce radical improvement in the ageing complexion. Recent studies suggest that AHAs may also act as free radical scavengers, sending messages to the dermis to increase collagen production and increase the skin's tolerance to retinoids.

### beauty spot

**Even at very low concentrations, AHAs can be irritating to some skins. If the normal initial tingling doesn't subside within a couple of minutes, or if your skin becomes visibly inflamed, refrain from using the product. It's possible a different product won't elicit the same response but if it does, console yourself with the knowledge that sunscreens are still a skin's best friend.**

### Collagen

It is used as an ingredient in cosmetics for its ability to hydrate and hold water on the skin, which in the skin's uppermost layers does very well. As a cosmetic ingredient, it has little effect on the skin's natural collagen which lies, beyond the remit of cosmetics, deep in the dermis.

### NMF

NMF is the skin's own moisturizer, made up of, among other, as yet undocumented ingredients, hyaluronic acid, a humectant with great water holding properties, urea, lactose, and amino acids. Frequent or harsh detergent washing, sun exposure and other environmental factors can deplete the skin's stores of NMF. It is the holy grail of many cosmetic scientists to be able to replicate the exact composition of NMF and put it into skin creams. To date, the best NMF is what your skin makes naturally. Hang on to it.

### Antioxidants

Usually included in skin creams in the form of vitamins A, C and E, they are capable of neutralizing the destructive effects of the free radical molecule. They do this by sacrificing electrons to free radicals before they get a chance to wrest one from a healthy cell.

The results of the 18-month SU.VI.MAX trial published in April 1998 suggest that not only do topically applied vitamins have a significantly protective effect, but that they can actually give your skin enough of a rest from fighting UV rays for it to achieve a degree of natural repair. Subjects who used the antioxidant cream showed a 2 per cent reduction in the depth of lines and wrinkles while the control group showed a 4 per cent increase in wrinkle depth.

### Humectants

These are substances which attract and hold moisture. They are useful in moisturizing cosmetic formulations for their ability to draw moisture from the air and hold it within the stratum corneum thereby helping to reduce water loss. Two humectants regularly used in cosmetic formulations are glycerine (a cheaper ingredient) and hyaluronic acid (a more expensive one).

### Lipids

This a generic term for a variety of fatty substances which constitute about 10 per cent of the stratum corneum, lipids fill the intercellular spaces sealing the skin's surface. Synthetic lipids are included in cosmetics in the hope that they will take the place of those removed by washing or destroyed by sun exposure and help to improve the barrier function.

### Retinoids

This is the generic term given to members of the vitamin A family which includes tretinoin, retinol, retinyl palmitate, retinyl acetate and retinyl propionate. Tretinoin (aka Retin-A) is the acid form of the molecule which clinical studies have shown to have the greatest level of activity in the rejuvenation of photo-damaged skin. It speeds up cell turnover bringing plump, new healthy skin cells to the surface more quickly, thereby smoothing out wrinkles and helping to clear acne. It is very irritating, however, and used only via prescription and under the supervision of a physician. Retinyl palmitate is much less irritating and so is often incorporated into cosmetic creams seeking a similar effect. However, it doesn't penetrate well or is never sufficiently well broken down by the skin to be of much benefit. Retinol is both slightly irritating and slightly effective. With careful adjustments to minimize irritation, it is now incorporated into a number of over-the-counter creams (eg RoC Retinol range and Estée Lauder Diminish).

## What are cosmeceuticals?

In the past, the distinction was clear: a cosmetic was a product for the beautification and enhancement of appearance; a drug was a preparation used to prevent or treat a disease. But today there exists a new hybrid – the cosmeceutical. It is a prescription pharmaceutical formulated to address a cosmetic problem.

Legally, however, the term cosmeceutical has yet to be recognized. While the Japanese authorities have created a new 'semi-drug' skin-care category, the United States' Food and Drug Administration, for example, as yet recognizes only minoxidil, the anti-baldness drug as a cosmeceutical. Prescription drugs which can be considered cosmeceuticals, however, include the alpha hydroxy acids (at concentrations of over 15 per cent), retinoic acid, and perhaps some of the ascorbates (vitamin C derivatives).

The trouble for the skin cream buying public is that many cosmetic companies are now using low concentrations of these same compounds. In so doing the companies face a choice. Either they provide clinical proof of the claim they make for their products and are forced to take it off the lucrative over-the-counter market. Or, they retain cosmetic status by not making any claims beyond the superficial. What most cosmetics companies have chosen to do is to sit resolutely on the fence. They are continuing to make and market preparations which, behind the closed doors of a press briefing or consultant training session, they insist have a rejuvenating effect. But in public, they claim nothing more than 'smoother, younger-feeling skin'. It's almost a complete reversal of the situation a decade ago when many cosmetics claimed infinitely more than they were capable of delivering.

In the current confusion, it is probably wise to obtain your cosmeceutical skin cream from a physician. He or she is best equipped to diagnose your skin's needs and tolerance levels. Happily, most cosmetics companies, keen not to frighten off customers who have become accustomed to the sweet-smelling, fabulous-feeling, innocuous wares, are limiting the activity levels of any new formulations.

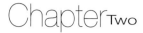

## Whole body skincare

**The care of body skin, with its fewer oil and more sweat glands, does differ. But for most people, skincare below the neck is a matter of controlling dryness.**

The most important thing about body skincare therefore is not to over cleanse and to bathe or shower in warm, not hot water, especially if your skin is very dry. In the past, skin was washed maybe once a week, but today, our keenness to eliminate all body odour and the need to soak away the strains of stressful modern living has meant that daily bathing or showering is now normal. While assiduous washing is good news for our neighbours' noses, it's not so good for our skin.

### Body hydration

Since the body's skin is almost always normal to dry, the liberal use of moisturizers is important. The best time to apply it is immediately after bathing while the skin is still damp. Doing so will lock in the moisture the skin has absorbed during the bath. Be sure to apply moisturizer very liberally to the arms and legs which can be especially dry. On areas such as elbows and heels, which if allowed to become especially dry can become painfully cracked, you might like to use a heavier cream (look for ones containing urea) or use one that contains an alpha hydroxy acid to refine the skin's outer layer.

If you like bathing or showering in the morning and have dry skin, be sure to apply cream or lotion before going to bed. The application of moisturizers at bedtime is more beneficial because the cream can be absorbed more in a warm bed.

If you have dry body skin it can often be improved by gentle exfoliation. The easiest way to do this is with a mildly abrasive cloth or by gently using a loofah. There are also many body exfoliating creams or cosmetic scrubs on the market. Which you use is both a matter of personal preference and how much you're prepared to spend. Body skin is less fragile than facial skin so physical exfoliation is fine. Again, as with facial skin, don't overdo it. If you experience increased dryness, smarting, burning or any form of irritation, you've overdone it.

As previously discussed, an alternative to physical exfoliation is to use a cream with an AHA to refine the outer skin layers. In some cosmetic preparations, AHAs are not present in sufficient concentration to make a marked difference to the look or feel of the skin and may be included as much for marketing as for skin smoothing reasons. Others, however, may have a significant effect – controlling both dryness and roughness.

### Hands

It is a fact that hands are the great 'give-aways' of age. According to our current understanding of the effects of UV rays, what they actually 'give away', of course, is the level of protection they have, or have not, received. Like our faces, our hands are constantly exposed to the elements but they receive far less care and attention, and are also subjected to much more rigorous tasks, including much more washing. Hence, hands may need as much, if not more, protection and moisture as our faces.

It's a good idea to keep a tube of SPF15 hand cream nearby, and to apply some whenever you feel the need. Moisturizer alone will stop the skin drying out, but it cannot prevent most of the ageing changes we so often see on hands: the so-called 'liver' spots which we now more correctly call age or sun spots, uneven pigmentation, thin, fragile-looking skin and lack of elasticity. Only a moisturizer with sun screen protection will do that.

*If you have dry skin, long soaks in hot baths should be avoided, particularly during the winter months as hot bath water can literally melt lipids from your skin. And if you wash with an alkaline soap and then lie in the sudsy water, the heat, alkaline salts in the water and soap surfactants will all conspire to rob your skin of protective lipids.*

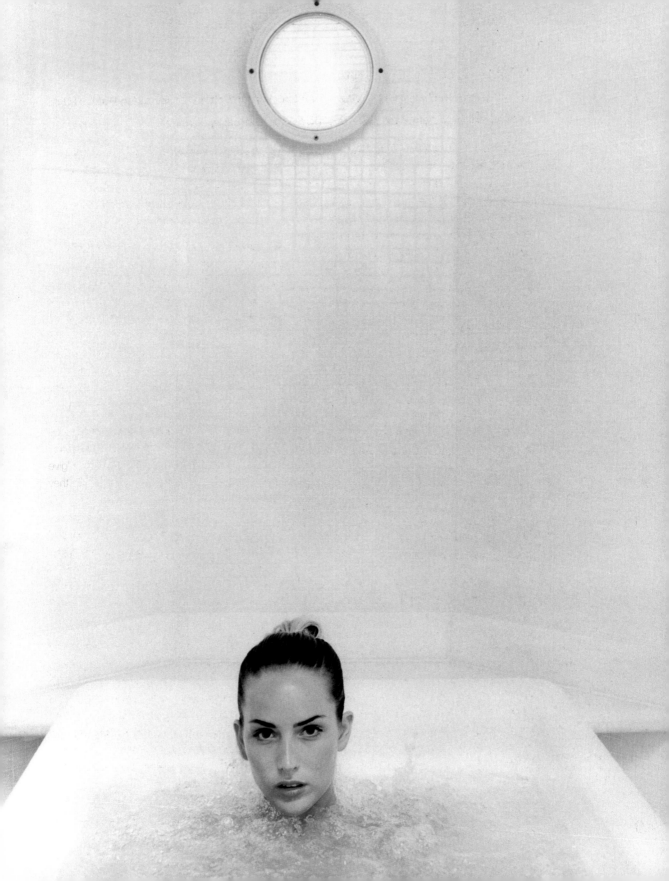

# 3 SUN: BURNING ISSUES AND PROTECTION RACKETS

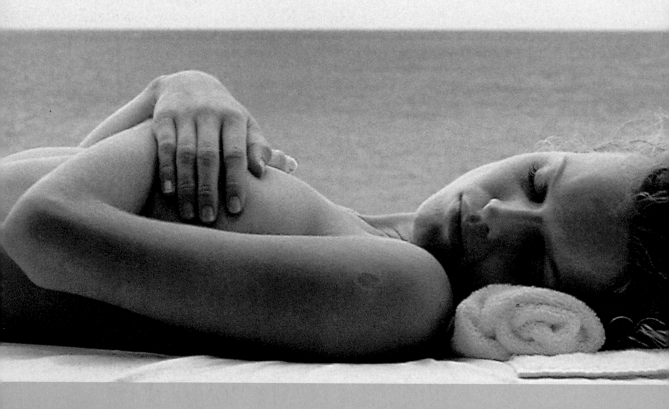

**Ultraviolet light has emerged as the most important factor in skin ageing. It is now beyond dispute that the rate and degree to which it wrinkles and sags, mottles or develops cancerous lesions depends largely on its level of exposure to UV rays.**

# Until Coco Chanel

famously stepped from a boat in St Tropez with her skin bronzed by the Mediterranean sun, milky skintones had been highly regarded in fashionable circles, largely because a tan marked out its possessor as a peasant who spent his or her days toiling in the fields. But well before Chanel set off on her cruise, tanned peasants were turning into pallid factory workers

## In the pursuit and maintenance of great-looking skin, protecting your skin from the sun is one of today's major health issues.

as the effects of the industrial revolution took hold. Tans were in. And they have remained in for most of this century.

However, once again, skin tone fashions are changing. The pace of change may be snail-slow when compared with the frenetic hems-up, hems-down gait of clothes fashions. But as we find out what the sun is really doing to our skin we are beginning to realise that tans are really not so attractive after all.

Britain's Health Education Authority (an organization which advises the government on

health issues), many magazine beauty editors and dermatologists are all currently engaged in attempting to persuade the public that a natural skin colour is best. It's working – in part. While not exactly eschewing tanning altogether, most people nowadays are more restrained in their sunbathing habits. The Health Education Authority, reports that 32 per cent of us have cut down on time spent sunbathing, and retailers report that rather than SPF 2s and 4s we are now buying SPF 15s.

But why exactly is that dermatologists, health and skincare experts tirelessly attempt to frighten you out of the sun entirely? How bad can it really be? Read on and decide for yourself.

### The ABC of sun damage

Solar radiation comprises short, high energy rays from cosmic, gamma and X to longer, lower energy ultraviolet, visible, infrared, micro- and radio waves all of which travel towards Earth at 300,000 kilometres per second in a straight but undulating line. Of those rays that pass through the atmosphere, it is only ultraviolet and infrared that are known to have a detrimental effect on the skin.

Ultraviolet rays range in wavelength from 190–400 nanometres. For convenience sake they are

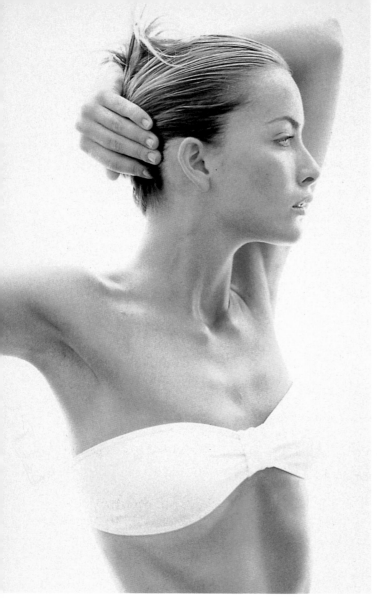

*Beautiful bodies remain that way for longer with the liberal use of high factor sunscreens.*

## UVB – the burning ray

The actions of UVB are manifold. On the surface of the skin, UVB peroxidizes our protective lipids, so compromising their barrier function. But the dehydrating effects are only the beginning. Only 20 per cent of UVB rays make it as far as the mid epidermis but those that do can 'cook' the cells there, turning some into big swollen pink mutants called sunburn cells and altering the molecular structure and nucleic proteins of others, predisposing them to cancerous mutations. This is sunburn. Sunburn isn't just the result of skin damage; it is in itself damaging. As the skin becomes inflamed, a more insidious form of injury takes place with the generation of rogue molecules called free radicals (see page 20). An unwelcome by-product of the normal cell oxidation process, the stress of sun exposure increases their production. What's more, free radical activity continues long after the sun goes down – for as long as the skin remains red and hot. Over time, UVB assaults your melanocytes beyond their ability to spread pigment evenly and they begin to dump clumps and clusters which show up as dark splodges.

## UVA – the ageing rays

Until last decade UVA rays were generally regarded as innocuous. But over the last fifteen years we have discovered that the shorter UVA rays are not only responsible for about 20 per cent of sunburn and can damage cellular DNA, but also that the longer UVA rays penetrate deep into the dermis where they cause the majority of the changes that we once associated with the

divided into three categories – A (340–400nm), B (320–340nm) and C (280nm and shorter).

Only those rays greater than 290nm reach the earth; UVC along with cosmic, gamma and X-rays are filtered out by the stratosphere, and UVC in particular by the ozone layer – happily, since it fatally mutates DNA. Ultraviolet and infra-red reach the earth's surface and penetrate our skin: UVB as far as our epidermis, UVA into the dermis and infrared right through to the subcutis.

natural ageing process. UVA intrusion into the dermis excites the cells there sufficiently to generate the production of the fearsome free radicals. Sensing danger, the body's immune system sends in repair enzymes – called, perfectly explicably if rather unimaginatively, collagense and elastase – which, mistaking an energy ray for a foreign invader begin to attack perfectly healthy collagen and elastin. Over time, the result of their repeated attack leaves collagen fibres weakened and elastin coils clumped into an inelastic mass. The visible effect of these microscopic changes are lines, wrinkles, dilated blood vessels where the dermis no longer holds firm the their walls and, in extreme cases, tough, waxy looking skin where blobs of toughened elastin rise from their dermal bed up into the epidermis. Even worse is the news of how little UVA it takes to severely damage your dermis.

### Why does UVB only burn sometimes while UVA always ages?

The amount of UVB that reaches the earth's surface varies with the season. A short, energetic ray, UVB doesn't travel great distances. It is therefore more plentiful during the summer months when the sun is more directly overhead. It is also easily blocked by cloud, clothing and even glass. UVA, however, is a longer, leaner ray. It doggedly rains down onto the earth's surface in both the summer and winter months. You may not, therefore, get burnt as you drive along in your air-conditioned car with all the windows closed, or sitting outside on a cloudy day, but you will certainly have soaked up plenty of ageing UVA rays.

### Infrared Rays

Infrared has been underestimated, not least because its effects fail to reveal themselves for decades. However, studies have shown that infrared destroys collagen, creates free radicals and causes the release of heat shock proteins which break down connective tissues, leading to an increased risk of skin ageing and cancers.

The time of day also affects the levels of A and B present. UVB rays only become a problem when the sun is high in the sky. They peak at about 12.30 and are all but exhausted by about 2 p.m. UVA, on the other hand, because it is closer in wavelength to visible light, is present almost all day.

UV radiation also increases with altitude. For every 300 metres (1,000 ft) you ascend there is a 4 per cent increase –which is why it is so important to adequately protect your skin during winter sports such as skiing and climbing.

## Delayed reactions

As anyone who's watched a ferocious sunburn flare up as the sun goes down knows, there is a delay between the time when sun damage is done and when it reveals itself. This hiatus has been carefully studied and documented.

- It takes up to eight hours for sunburn from UVB rays to become visible. (24 hours for UVA)
- Redness and discomfort peaks around 20 hours later. (After 48 hours for UVA)
- It will be up to 48 hours before the sunburn subsides. (72 hours for UVA)

Why there is a delay isn't fully understood but it is thought that the injury is sufficient to temporarily subdue the skin's defence and repair mechanisms. Whatever the reason, it is important to keep this period of calm-before-the-storm in mind when sunbathing: failure to do so can be painful in the short term and in the long term will affect the appearance and health of your skin.

# Chapter Three

## Your skin under the sun

**When it comes to withstanding the effects of the sun, all skins are not created equal.**

**The amount of melanin your skin produces determines your level of natural protection.**

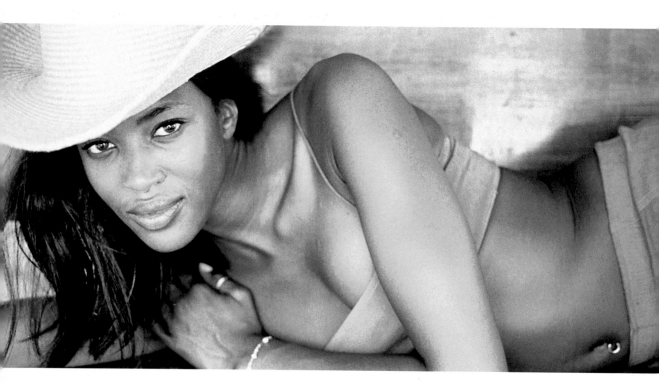

*Black, white or red all over? How your resistant your skin is to the sun's rays depends on the quantity and quality of melanin it produces.*

In his book *Self-Made Man and his Undoing*, anthropologist Jonathan Kingdon concludes that humans probably began life with a mid-brown colour and that black and white skins developed as a result of the environmental conditions that people had to live with. Black skin was necessary for people living in the equatorial regions to survive the constant ultraviolet assault. Those who moved north could forgo sun protection in favour of the more efficient vitamin D production that comes with paler skin. (Dark skin inhibits vitamin D production, which is why rickets, the bone disease, was so common in people of African origin who moved to northern countries.)

What is surprising about different skin colours is that whatever our race, everyone has roughly the same number of melanocytes, the pigment producing cells of your epidermis. The difference lies in the quantity, and quality, of melanin each melanocytes produces. A dark, sticky, treacly substance, melanin forms a physical shield over the cells nucleus to help protect DNA. It absorbs and reflects UV rays and is also a fabulously efficient free radical scavenger.

### beauty spot

**Sunscreens are only part of a sensible 'safe sun' plan. You also need to:**

- **Wear protective clothing such as hats and long-sleeved shirts**

- **Seek shade between the hours of 11am and 3pm. If you have very fair skin, extend this period from 10am to 4pm.**

## Your skin in the sun

| Skin type | Response to sun | Characteristics | Natural tan SPF (approximate) |
|---|---|---|---|
| 1 | Burns badly, may freckle but never tans. Any colour gained is more red than brown. High cancer risk | Celtic types – pale skin; often freckled; normally blue or green eyes; blonde, dark (Irish) or red hair | SPF 1.0 |
| 2 | Burns readily, tans slightly – tan will be light and reddish gold. High cancer risk | Fair skin, possibly freckled; light coloured eyes; blondes, redheads, or dark haired if of Irish extraction | SPF 1.5 |
| 3 | Burns first, tans gradually – tan is golden brown. Moderate cancer risk | The vast majority of Europeans and North Americans of European extraction, some light Asians; various eye and hair colour | SPF 2.5 |
| 4 | Burns minimally, tans well – skin colour is rich 'milk chocolate' brown. Low cancer risk, high risk of brown patches | Hispanic and Asian and the darker Mediterranean types; hair and eyes almost always brown | SPF 4.0 |
| 5 | Burns rarely, tans deeply – dark chocolate shade. Very low cancer risk, high risk of brown patches | Far Eastern, Indian, Polynesian | SPF 6.5 |
| 6 | Almost never burns, but does darken. Extremely low cancer risk | African, African-American, West Indian | SPF 9.0 |
| 7 | Unlikely to burn. Extremely low cancer risk | Central Aftrican, Australian Aborigine | SPF 10.0 |

The best quality melanin, as mentioned previously, is eumelanin (2). It is thick, almost black and viscous. Phaeomelanin on the other hand is yellowish (in Asian skins) or reddish-brown (in Celtic skins) in colour and is neither as good at deflecting ultraviolet rays nor of mopping up free radicals. Very dark black skins, as you might imagine, produce masses of the black variety of melanin – about 400 melanosomes, or pockets or melanin per basal epidermal cell – while very white skins produce 30 times less, and most of it is the inferior phaeomelanin.

In addition to this 30-fold increased protection of the epidermis, black skin inhibits the passage of UVA into the dermis up to five times better than white skin. Not only do black skins not burn as readily, therefore, they also don't suffer as much from the 'premature ageing' that often afflicts white skins.

# Your skin's own defence strategy

**Despite red hot evidence to the contrary, your skin is actually remarkably well equipped to deal with the damaging effects of UV rays. But then again, the sun is responsible for much more than sunburn and premature ageing – happily not all of it negative.**

Reading through the catalogue of sun-induced skin changes, you could be forgiven for concluding that our flesh is about as useful in defending us from ultraviolet attack as a silk slip is in stopping bullets. In fact, our skin is extraordinarily capable both of fending off attack and of repairing much of the injury inflicted. For the most part, it performs an exemplary life-long role of protecting us from the outside world. That it becomes wrinkled and blotched in the process is, in evolutionary terms, neither here nor there. Wrinkles and age spots don't kill, nor do they ever seriously affect our general health. If wrinkles were a life threatening condition, you can be sure that evolution would be working on weeding them out. Even skin cancers, the incidence of which is, worryingly, steadily rising, are rarely a problem before our sixth or seventh decade. Until a few years ago we couldn't reasonably expect to live long enough to see skin cancer develop, let alone see it endanger our lives.

There are a number of complex mechanisms by which our skin protects itself from ultraviolet rays, the very first of which is sebum. Some UVB rays don't even get past our oily outer mantle because sebum itself blocks them – another reason why oily skins are better equipped to cope with the sun. What does get through

### beauty spot

**Hidden Melanin: although your 'tan line' may indicate otherwise, melanin production isn't limited to exposed areas of skin. A study reported in the journal *Management of Wilderness and Environmental Emergencies*, demonstrated melanin production in unexposed areas, too – presumably a peremptory safeguard against you one day deciding to swap your one-piece for a bikini.**

induces skin to protect itself by a) thickening and by b) tanning.

### Thick skin

After several days of UVB exposure, your stratum corneum thickens considerably – up to six times its normal depth. If you are still horrified by the seeming inadequacy of your skin to cope with the sun you may be reassured to know that a well thickened stratum corneum absorbs or reflects up to 75 per cent of UVB. (This thickening does not occur with UVA irradiation which is why sunbeds are not a worthwhile pre-holiday prophylactic measure.) Because they are almost dead anyway, anucleic, keratin-filled stratum corneum cells are relatively unaffected by the UVB they absorb.

NB: You should be aware that if you use active skincare products which are formulated to smooth and refine the stratum corneum (eg AHAs and retinol or retinoid-based creams) you will be removing some of this natural protection. You should therefore be particularly assiduous in your use of sunscreen.

### Tanned hide

As and when the ultraviolet light frazzles a section of DNA, excisor enzymes are dispatched to snip out the botched bit and make way for a perfect new piece. The duplicate piece which arrives to take its place is called a thymine dimer. It is the presence of this dimer which sparks the melanocytes into action. Melanocyte stimulating hormone (MSH), which is already circulating, waiting for the call up, begins to bind to the melanocytes. The spiky arms of these dentritic cells grow and branch out, each eventually touching about 36 keratinocytes. Then tyrosine, the melanin pre-cursor is brought into play and, courtesy of various enzymes, is turned into melanin. Pockets of melanin are incorporated into organelles called melanosomes and then packed off to take up residence in the surrounding keratinocytes (epidermal cells). There they form a physical umbrella over the cell nucleus to prevent radiation falling on the DNA and RNA. Some melanosomes, meanwhile, hang around in the spaces between cells to help mop up pillaging free radicals.

Neither toughening nor tanning happens immediately. It takes several days of repeated exposure for your outer layer of skin to build up, 36 hours for the first of your melanin to be produced and about three weeks before it is reaches its protective plateau – something to remember on the first few days of your holiday.

Both of the above defence mechanisms concern the epidermis only. It is reasonable that the skin puts its most determined efforts into fighting UVB (and short wave UVA). After all, only they can cause life-threatening, cancerous changes. It does mean, however, that you will have to step in to protect your skin from longer, prematurely ageing UVA rays.

Further damage limitation occurs in both epidermis and dermis in the form of free radical scavenging. A number of natural anti-oxidants (superoxidedismutase, glutathione, melanin) are on hand, ready and willing to sacrifice bits of themselves to free radicals generated by the sun. These naturally-occurring anti-oxidants are extraordinarily powerful. However, they are very quickly exhausted by ultraviolet radiation – after twenty minutes of exposure, levels of glutathione, for instance have markedly fallen. The more we find out about how good natural anti-oxidants are, and about how quickly they are used, the more skincare companies are attempting to build extracted or synthesized versions into their sun and after-sun products. As you will have read in other chapters, free radical scavengers, natural or topically-applied, are fast becoming thought of as key weapons in the fight against skin damage.

When you are young your skin's defence and repair mechanisms work at full efficiency. But as you age, its ability to keep up with the maintenance programme slows. There comes a point when, if the level of damage exceeds the potential for repair, regeneration turns to degeneration. This is the point when UV damage begins to accumulate, the end result of which is weathered, wrinkled skin.

## Beyond sunburn

The sun is a well-known immune system depressant. So, despite the fact you go on holiday feeling healthy, you can sometimes develop an unattractive cold sore, for example. The reason for this is that ultraviolet rays damage the tentacles of the Langerhan's cells, the immune system's spiky sentries.

**Skin aggravation** There are other conditions which may be aggravated by the sun including acne, rosacea (see Chapter 5) and lupus erythematosus. If you experience a flare-up of an existing skin condition in the sun, conceal the area under clothing and use high factor sun protection on other exposed areas. On your return see a dermatologist.

**Polymorphic light eruption** This is often incorrectly called 'prickly heat' but PLE is an allergic-type reaction to the UVA sun rays. It is suffered by up to 14 per cent of the white population, 60–70 per cent of them female. True prickly heat is not sun-induced but occurs in hot, humid conditions when the sweat glands overwork and become blocked. Distinguishing PLE from prickly heat is relatively easy; the PLE rash generally occurs in sun-exposed areas while prickly heat is found where the sun rarely reaches – in skin creases like armpits and groin.

The skin reaction usually occurs one to five days after first severe sun exposure and it usually happens on skin that hasn't seen the sun for some time. You can help to prevent PLE with a high-factor, broad-spectrum sunscreen. But once a PLE rash has flared up it will take 7–10 days to subside, provided it is covered. You might be tempted to assume the rash is due to a reaction to your sunscreen – understandable given it usually occurs where you apply cream – but the safety of modern formulations means this is rarely the case.

## Super sun-sensitive skin

Certain drugs and chemicals when applied to the skin or ingested can heighten your skin's susceptibility to UV-damage.

**Retin-A** (also known as tretinoin or retinoic acid), the anti-acne, and anti-wrinkle drug, is perhaps the best known sun sensitizer. As you can read in Chapter 5 and Chapter 7 retinoic acid is a vitamin A acid preparation with the ability to dramatically speed up the epidermal cell turnover rate resulting in a finer, clear, spot-free and less wrinkled complexion. But this refined complexion doesn't offer the same protection as a thick one so physicians prescribing Retin-A (it is only available on prescription) are careful to recommend, if not insist, that their patients use a minimum of SPF15 all day, every day.

**Other compounds** Psoralen plant chemicals,

some metal compounds such as arsenic, scents including those containing musk, and certain drugs can also cause your skin to become very sensitive to the sun. Ferocious burns can occur from just mild exposure.

Psoralens are thought to work by inducing changes in the DNA and RNA structure, which in turn alters their UV-absorption spectrum. The most notorious psoralen is bergamot, the small citrus fruit whose extract was included in, and gave its name to, Bergasol sun products – it also flavours Earl Grey tea.

**Drug-induced sensitivities** A wide series of drugs can cause problems in the sun.

● Antibiotics such as tetracycline and doxycycline.
● Drugs used to treat urinary tract infections such as ciprofloxacillin and nalidixic acid.
● Arthritis medications such as feldene and naprosyn.
● Diuretics such as thiazides.
● Antihistamines such as diphenhydreamine (as in Benadryl – which may be of particular interest to sunbathing hay fever sufferers).

It is thought that these drugs affect the structure of the cell membrane making it more prone to absorb higher doses of UV rays.

In practical terms what you will see is a very exaggerated burn, severe redness perhaps accompanied by blistering, and change in pigmentation. Unfortunately, the burn may not show up for 24 to 72 hours after exposure as the injury inflicted vastly increases the normal delay times.

**Environmental risks** Certain chemicals in our environment are phototoxic – that is combined with ultraviolet rays they become poisonous and in some cases cause damage to DNA. These

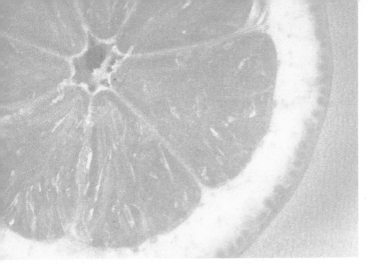

*If splashed on the skin, the natural chemicals contained in some citrus fruits can intensify the effects of the sun.*

**Good dietary sources** For those at risk, milk, eggs, cereals, margarine, and oily fish (such as salmon, herring and mackerel), for example, contain good levels of vitamin D. A bowl of cereal will supply about half your necessary daily allowance while half a 200g tin of salmon will give you 13mcg, 8 mcg more than the recommended daily allowance.

## Treating skin diseases

In about 80 per cent of cases, patients who are suffering from psoriasis, eczema, acne and vitiligo will experience some improvement in their condition after exposure to ultraviolet radiation. (See also Chapter 6). But the dose needs to be carefully managed by a dermatologist to ensure the maximum benefit with minimum damage.

## Seasonal affective disorder (SAD)

Sufferers of this condition experience depression because of the lack of light during the short winter days. However, it is the lack of visible light entering the body that is to blame for the condition, not the absence of UV. Sufferers who use sun lamps, which emit visible wavelengths, to alleviate their condition will not be compromising their skin.

---

include arsenic, petrochemicals and benzene dyes. These chemicals directly damage cellular DNA throughout the body and can predispose cells to cancerous changes.

## The good news – at last

Don't despair – although most of the effects of the sun's ultraviolet rays are indeed negative to our skin, there are also a few benefits that we derive from them. The rays produce vitamin D, help improve skin conditions such as acne and psoriasis, and can help seasonal affective disorder (SAD) sufferers.

## Vitamin D production

Vitamin D is vital for a healthy skeleton because it works with calcium to help form strong bones. Although you can get adequate amounts of vitamin D by eating a healthy diet, an important source of vitamin D is sunlight. A vitamin D deficiency in children can lead to the 'bendy bone' deformity called rickets, while in adults it can contribute to osteomalacia (bone softening) or osteoporosis (reduction in bone density leading to brittle bones). But this doesn't mean you can stop using a sunscreen, because a pale-skinned person with just a bit of skin exposed will produce sufficient vitamin D for several days after just 10 minutes in spring or summer sunshine.

---

Psoralens are mainly found in:

- citrus fruits (*Rutaceae* family) including limes, lemon, citron, bitter orange and bergamot (Also in common rue.)
- lichens
- many of the plants and weeds which grow wild in gardens and pastures including buttercup, giant hogweed, celery, parsnip, fennel, yarrow, bindweed, carrot and dill.
- figs

A psoralen-induced sunburn makes your skin darker, redder and more painful, and so therefore last longer.

# Chapter Three

## Sunscreening - how, when and with what

**Enjoying the psychological benefits of sunshine and keeping your skin in the style to which you're accustomed need not be mutually exclusive. Modern sunscreens are formulated to offer protection against the full spectrum of damaging rays.**

### Getting blanket protection

The first commercial sunscreens, which came onto the US market in 1928, were based on chemicals that absorbed the energy of UVB rays. These were developed solely with the aim of preventing burning: neither the existence nor effect of UVA was yet known. Indeed, by the seventies – the days of baby oil and tin-foil reflectors, of mahogany jet-setters and quick-tan competitions – it seemed the only reason to wear sun creams was so that you could avoid a sunburn so painful it might keep you from roasting yourself further. The beautiful people sported skins the colour of antique furniture and anyone who dared expose a piece of flesh paler than a deli-cabinet roasted chicken was rewarded with snorts of derision.

**beauty spot**

Antioxidants are often used in sunscreens, the idea being that any free radicals generated by the odd UV rays that do get through will be quenched before they do any damage. Indeed, although not currently accepted as photoprotective agents in their own right, some experts are beginning to think of antioxidants as essential sunscreen ingredients.

A decade later, the effects of the searing seventies could be seen in the rising incidence of skin cancer, (up 90 per cent between 1974 and 1989). Greater attention was focused on cutting out the short UVB wave that caused it. Then, it was thought if you could inhibit burning but allow the passage of UVA you could induce a safe tan. 'The short-term aim of the sunbather,' wrote John V Simmons in *The Science of Cosmetics* (volume 1 of *Science and the Beauty Business*), 'is a rapid tan with no sunburn. The sunscreen they require is one which ideally would let through UV-A but not UV-B.' And so sunscreen manufacturers triumphantly launched products which they claimed were the solutions to the sunbather's conundrum. One brand's advertisement, for example, promised simply, 'turns ultra-violet into ultra-brown'.

But, of course, a sunscreen which lets through UVA also allows the acceleration of the ageing process, and possibly also the formation of skin cancers. By the mid 1980s, skincare companies which spent millions on researching and developing creams to keep skin looking young and beautiful were scrabbling around for UVA filters to put in their face-saving preparations. But filtering out UVA is no easy task – most UVB filters have little or no effect on A. Casting around for ways to combat UVA, scientists looked again at the physical sun blockers.

Zinc oxide and titanium dioxide pastes had long been known to obstruct the sun's rays. The advantage of physical reflectors over chemical absorbers is two-fold. Firstly, physical blockers reflect the sun's rays equally and secondly, they are inert and so, unlike some chemical filters, won't induce irritant reactions. The cosmetic catch, however, was that these compounds are opaque. Cricketers who spend all day in the outfield are happy to sport white stripes, but the gilded goddesses sunning themselves on the Club 55 beach in St Tropez are not. For them, the solution came in the form of the micronized particle. If you take zinc oxide and titanium dioxide and mill it down to a fine powder which you then blend into a cream or lotion, it's possible to get an almost invisible physical barrier.

*Dark skins have a natural protection factor of about 10 but are still not immune to the effects of UV rays.*

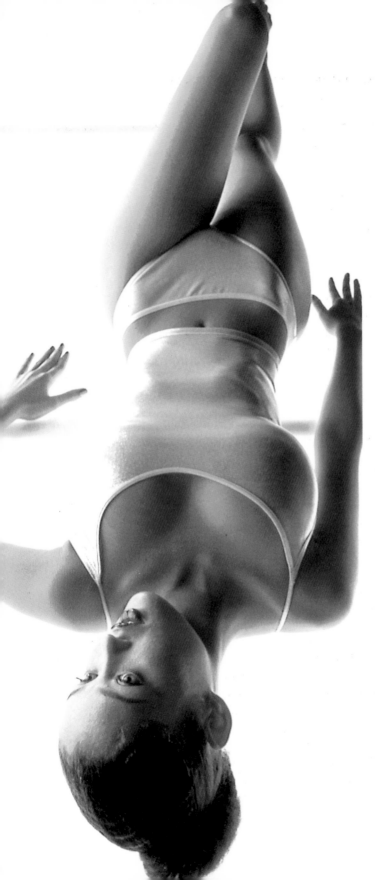

# sun: burning issues

Today, the most efficient sunscreens are those which offer broad spectrum protection – that is, that block or filter out UVA, UVB and infrared rays. New chemicals capable of absorbing UVA have recently been developed (eg Parsol 1789) but often sunscreen manufacturers can best achieve blanket protection by concocting a blend of chemical absorbers and physical blockers.

## Deciphering the labels
### Know your SPFs

Contrary to popular opinion a preparation's SPF (Sun Protection Factor) doesn't tell you the amount of time you can spend in the sun without getting burnt but the amount of extra time. For instance, if your skin normally burns after 20 minutes, an SPF8 means you can expect to inhibit burning for 20 x 8, ie for 2 hours and 40 minutes. SPF20 would prevent burning for over 6 hours.

### SPF – how high can you go?

SPF15 blocks out about 93 per cent of UVB and SPF20 about 97 per cent. You might think that there's little to choose between the two. Certainly the Australian authorities thought as much and restricted the labelling of sunscreens to a maximum of SPF15. In the US, where there is no such restriction, SPF32, 60 and upwards are not unheard of. However, recent findings have shown that the extra 4 per cent protection offered by SPF20 may well be significant in the prevention of skin cancers and it is currently being proposed that the upper limit be raised.

**Broad spectrum** means that the cream screens out both UVA and UVB. It does not, however, give you any indication of the degree of protection offered.

**Vitamins A, C and E** means that the cream contains antioxidant vitamins designed to help neutralize free radicals.

## Can sunscreens cause cancer?

Every spring for the last few years newspapers have carried stories stating: 'Sunscreens cause skin cancer'. The stories are based either on concerns that UVB sunscreens which prevent your skin from burning may be allowing you to soak up large doses of potentially cancer-causing UVA without your knowledge or on new findings suggesting that some sunscreen ingredients may actually be intrinsically damaging to skin cells. Much more work is needed in this later area but in the meantime keep in mind that it is unwise to rely solely on sunscreens; we should learn to avoid the sun, stay in the shade and cover up.

## UVA protection – how do you know what you're getting?

In order to get good, broad spectrum protection, chemists usually have to use a mixture of chemical and physical filters. But how can you tell what they've put into a cream and what sort of protective mix you're getting?

*With high factor, broad spectrum, waterproof sunscreens, sun and fun need not be mutually exclusive.*

In 1992, frustrated by the absence of a universally-recognized UVA rating system, Boots the Chemists in Britain, which sells 48 per cent of sunscreen products, launched its Star System. It decreed that suppliers would have to detail their preparation's level of UVA protection. If it filtered out as much UVA as UVB it achieved a maximum rating of four stars. If it filtered only 75 per cent as much A as B, it got three stars and so on down.

The system has now been running for six years and generally

### beauty spot

**In Britain, a government survey revealed that 24 per cent of those questioned thought the SPF figure stood for the number of minutes you could stay in the sun without burning, 16 per cent thought it represented the number of minutes you should apply the cream before going into the sun, and 6 per cent thought it related to the age group for whom the screen was best suited.**

has been welcomed by consumers and healthcare experts alike. So when choosing a sunscreen in Britain, choose your SPF first according to skin type – the higher the better – and then look for four stars for efficient protection against sun burn, skin cancer and premature ageing. Elsewhere in the world, unfortunately, you will have to put your trust in the name on the bottle.

## How to wear your sunscreen

You might think this paragraph redundant but 50 per cent of us rarely wear enough sun cream to get the full SPF printed on the bottle. If you buy an SPF20, but use an insufficient amount you may only achieve an SPF of 15 or even 10. You need to use a minimum of a teaspoonful over your face and neck. A dessertspoonful for each arm and more than a tablespoonful for each leg.

You also need to apply it soon enough. Chemical filters, particularly, need time to bind well to the skin so you should apply your cream to dry skin about 20 minutes before exposure. (If you apply it to wet or sweaty skin it will rub off easily leaving you unprotected.) And remember to reapply your cream often.

If you are swimming or playing sports you will need a water or sweat-proof formulation not only because your protection may wash away, but also because UV rays actually penetrate below the water's surface.

## Protecting children

Anecdotal evidence has long suggested that short, sharp sun burn shocks in childhood (or indeed later) can increase your risk of developing skin cancer. A recent Australian study appears to confirm this. It showed that those who moved to Australia as children had a higher incidence of skin cancer than those who had moved to Australia as adults.

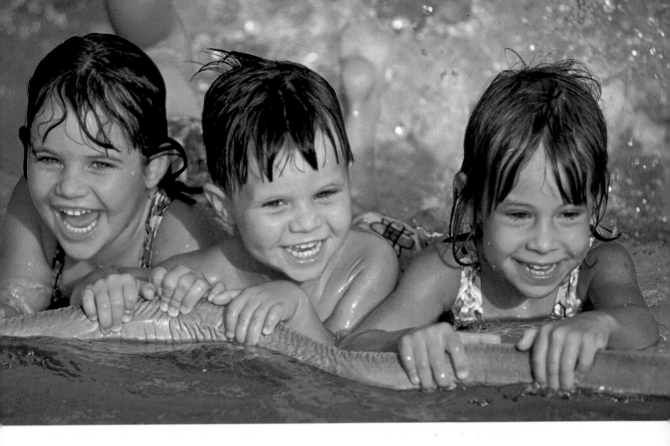

## Crisis management

Whatever the cause, if you or your child finishes the day red and sore, there are emergency measures you can take to limit the damage. Sunburn can be serious, especially if it is coupled with dehydration. The dual effect can cause chills, fever, shaking and swelling in the burnt areas.

In a child under the age of about 10, the effects can be exaggerated. A badly burnt shivering child should be taken to hospital immediately as he or she may need specialist treatment including intravenous rehydration. Severe sunburn which blisters should also be seen by a physician as the open sores can become infected.

Less severe cases can be treated as follows:

- Drink plenty of water. You and your skin are likely to be dehydrated, especially if your sunburn is the result of drinking in the sun and forgetting about protection.
- Take aspirin or ibuprofen to help reduce the inflammation.
- Use cold compresses on burnt areas to help bring down the temperature of the skin.
- Eat plenty of fresh fruit and vegetables containing vitamins A, C and E to help offset the destructive free radical rampage. You could also take a mega 1500 mg dose vitamin C supplement as any shock to your system rapidly depletes vitamin C stocks.

## Faking it

There is one safe tan – but it has to be fake. Those who haven't tried fake tans since they last found themselves adorned in tangerine stripes and veiled in an unpleasant smell, will doubtless be pleasantly surprised by the new generation of self-tanners.

A slight smell persists but is concealed by masking scents. And thanks to the discovery that the active ingredient in almost all self-tanners, DHA (dihydroxyacetone) turns brown in an acid environment but orange in an alkaline one, the colour they now impart is truly a 'tan' tan.

Many manufacturers now add fruit acids to their preparation to both improve the colour and keep it even and smooth.

### Which product?

There is a wide variety of self-tanners on the market – creams and lotions, gels and sprays. There is very little to choose between them. I (Polly) have tried them all. I've even painted many different stripes on a model's stomach in an attempt to tell them apart. Neither those of us in the studio, nor the camera could. The tonal differences were at best minimal. Probably the best way, therefore, is to choose your self-tanner by price and/or texture.

### beauty spot

Even if a bottle of fake tan states an SPF remember that this protection will last only a few hours while the tan itself will last several days. However, there is now some suggestion that the stain of a fake tan may inhibit the penetration of the longer UVA ray. Researchers who applied a 15 per cent DHA self-tanner to psoriasis patients undergoing Psoralen UVA therapy found that self-tanned skin showed less UVA-damage.

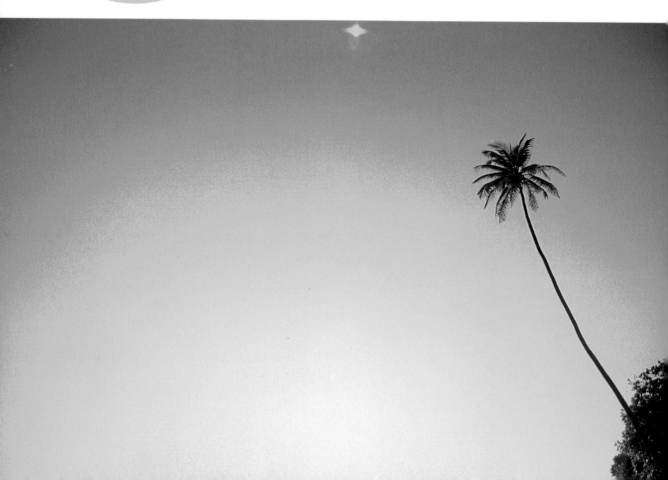

## How to apply a fake tan

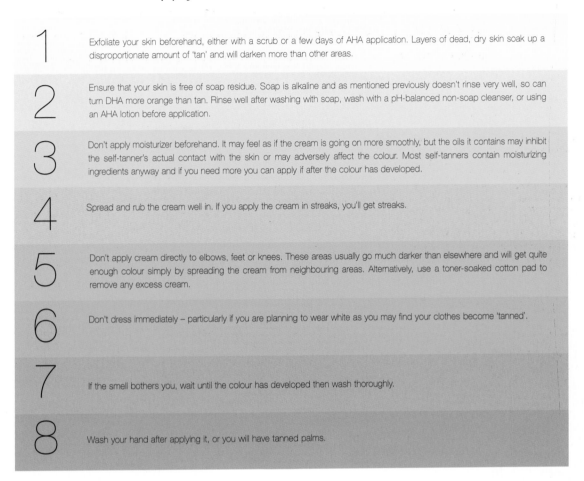

**1** Exfoliate your skin beforehand, either with a scrub or a few days of AHA application. Layers of dead, dry skin soak up a disproportionate amount of 'tan' and will darken more than other areas.

**2** Ensure that your skin is free of soap residue. Soap is alkaline and as mentioned previously doesn't rinse very well, so can turn DHA more orange than tan. Rinse well after washing with soap, wash with a pH-balanced non-soap cleanser, or using an AHA lotion before application.

**3** Don't apply moisturizer beforehand. It may feel as if the cream is going on more smoothly, but the oils it contains may inhibit the self-tanner's actual contact with the skin or may adversely affect the colour. Most self-tanners contain moisturizing ingredients anyway and if you need more you can apply if after the colour has developed.

**4** Spread and rub the cream well in. If you apply the cream in streaks, you'll get streaks.

**5** Don't apply cream directly to elbows, feet or knees. These areas usually go much darker than elsewhere and will get quite enough colour simply by spreading the cream from neighbouring areas. Alternatively, use a toner-soaked cotton pad to remove any excess cream.

**6** Don't dress immediately – particularly if you are planning to wear white as you may find your clothes become 'tanned'.

**7** If the smell bothers you, wait until the colour has developed then wash thoroughly.

**8** Wash your hand after applying it, or you will have tanned palms.

### It's never too late

If you have misspent your youth staked out under the sun, the news that the sun has mutated your DNA, deflated your dermis and coagulated your melanin won't be welcome. You probably feel that having missed the 'prevention boat' you must now resign yourself to growing old with a disgraceful complexion or embarking on a series of costly cures. Think again.

In recent years it has become apparent that the skin's extraordinary recuperative powers can undo some of the damage done. In 1982 Dr Lorraine Kligman at the University of Pennsylvania, showed that skin which was fully protected by ultraviolet light actually grew new dermal collagen within ten weeks. And in Australia, researchers revealed that subjects who applied a sunscreen every morning during the Australian summer developed fewer skin pre-cancers than in previous years and any existing solar keratoses actually regressed. Both studies demonstrated that, when given the chance, sun damaged skin can affect a degree of natural repair.

*The burning UVB ray is at the peak of its power at noon during summer months, but the ageing UVA rays beat down summer and winter, rain and shine.*

# 4 HAIR AND NAILS

**You may be wondering why hair and nails are included in a book about skin. It's because your hair and nails are an extension of skin. Both grow from the same epidermal tissue which makes skin cells, and both consist largely of the protein keratin.**

# nine weeks after

you are conceived, the first hairs on your eyebrows, upper lip and chin are actually established. By the time you are a 16-week old foetus, you will have an estimated 5 million hair follicles, of which only about 100,000 are located on your scalp.

In fact, apart from the palms of your hands, the soles of your feet and your lips, you have hair follicles over all your body. Some produce long,

## How curly or straight, wavy or fine your hair is depends on the size and shape of the hair follicle.

thick coloured hairs such as on the scalp, others produce shorter coloured ones such as those on your eyebrows, in your pubic and underarm areas and in men's beards, but the majority grow tiny, fine translucent ones, called vellus hairs, such as those over your cheeks or stomach.

Whether thick and dark or fine and fair, each hair is similar in construction. The shaft consists of several concentric layers of elongated keratin protein cells which are formed in the bulbous part of the follicle deep in the dermis. The inner layer of the shaft is the medulla – the living core – although this may not be present, at least not all the way through the

hair shaft. Its role is not clearly understood. The middle layer is the cortex which also contains pockets (melanocytes) of melanin pigment, which as in your skin, gives your hair its protection and colour. The outer layer is the cuticle which comprises five to ten layers of overlapping sheets, or curved tiles, of keratinocyte cells. Composed of anucleic cells, all hairs are essentially 'dead' matter.

### The cuticle – the key to glossy hair

The examination under a microscope of glossy hair would reveal that each hair shaft was covered in tightly-bound, overlapping layers of keratinoyctes. When the layers lie flat and close over one another, light bounces evenly off each individual hair shaft making your hair look fabulously shiny. Just as successful skin-care depends on keeping your stratum corneum clear, clean and intact, so successful hair care depends on keeping your cuticle the same.

**beauty spot**
**The number of hair follicles you have is genetically-determined and neither increases nor decreases after birth. It doesn't matter what you do to your head or body hair – shave it, wax it, pluck it or dye it – you cannot cause more hair to grow. It is what occurs within your body, including fluctuating hormone, nutrition and temperature levels, that can affect the type and rate of hair growth.**

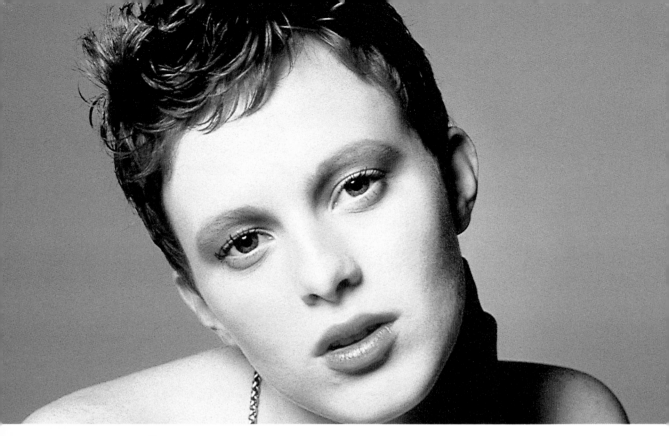

## The long and the short of it

Hair grows in cycles of three phases; a growing anogen phase, a transitional catogen phase, and finally a resting telogen phase. Then the hair falls out and the cycle begins again. The length of your particular cycle is genetic and how long your hair will grow depends on how long its anogen phase is. As most hair grows about half an inch a month, someone with a six-year anogen phase could grow hair three feet long whilst someone with a two-year growing phase could only grow two feet of hair. As you get older, the growing phase gets shorter and the resting phase longer meaning that even if you wanted to, past the age of fifty, you probably couldn't grow hair past your waist.

## Hair loss – what's normal?

There are about 100,000 hairs on your scalp, each follicle going through its 1,000 day cycle (about 20 times a lifetime). The number of hairs you naturally lose a day depends on your cycle but anything from 25 to 100 hairs a day is completely normal. If you are concerned about excessive hair loss, see Chapter 6 for possible causes and solutions.

## The curly and the straight

How curly or straight, wavy or fine your hair is depends on the size and shape of the follicle from which the hair grows. Oriental hair grows from the large circular follicles, African hair is the product of a 'crinkle-cut' oval-shaped follicle and Caucasian hair runs the gamut inbetween. The size and shape of your hair follicles are genetically determined but the texture of your hair can change over time. The reason some people's straight hair becomes curly at adolescence is thought to occur when, as a result of accelerated growth, the follicle moves deeper into the dermis, twisting as it does so and forcing the hair to corkscrew out from it.

### The black and the blonde

Your natural hair colour is controlled in part by the same pigment responsible for your skin colour – melanin. As you have read in Chapter 3, there are two different shades of melanin: eumelanin, which is brown to black, and phaeomelanin which is yellow to red. In hair there is also a third type, oxymelanin, also yellow to red, which is a naturally bleached version of eumelanin.

### Going, going grey

If you are going grey and not enjoying the experience, it is doubly depressing to discover that the reason for loss of hair colour is not yet fully understood and, as a result, there are no imminent cures. What is apparent is that the ability of the melanocytes to produce pigment declines with the years. Perhaps they become exhausted earlier than other parts of our bodies because they work so hard. The hair bulb is an area of some of the most intense cellular proliferation seen anywhere in our bodies. Most Caucasians begin to see their first white hairs by their mid thirties while in black races the onset of grey comes a decade later.

The loss of colour is not the only problem. Many people complain that their previously sleek, perfectly behaved hair becomes wiry and unmanageable as it greys. Lack of melanin not only means hair is less protected from UV damage, but also less able to retain its optimum moisture levels. Using sunscreening hair products, good conditioners and availing yourself of the wealth of sleekening styling preparations now available (look for ones with silicone in them), will help avoid the unflattering 'wire wool' look.

## The key to glossy hair

As you have read, ultimately, great-looking glossy hair is dependent on a tightly packed cuticle.

### You can keep your cuticle flat by:

- washing your hair regularly – preferably once a day – to maintain your hair's water balance. When moisture is lost the outer cells of the layers of cuticle tend to curl up, resulting in duller, drier-looking hair
- using conditioner to smooth down the scales and lock in the necessary moisture
- towelling your hair dry by squeezing rather than rubbing
- using silicone serums to help detangle your hair easily
- never brushing your hair, but using a wide-toothed comb when it is wet, gently beginning at the bottom and working upwards in sections
- using sunscreening hair products.

### You can ruffle your cuticle by:

- washing with harsh detergents or alkaline soap
- vigorous towel drying
- handling it roughly, particularly when wet
- having your hair permed or bleached which by its very nature opens the cuticle to break down proteins bonds or leech out pigment
- using very hot styling devices too long and too often
- letting it get sunburnt.

## Washing instructions

'How to' directions on the back of a shampoo bottle on how to wash your hair may seem as unnecessary as 'how to walk' instructions on a new pair of shoes, but according to trichologist Dr Hugh Rushton, there are many myths surrounding hair washing, (for instance: washing in cold water increases shine). His advice for correct hair cleansing and conditioning is as follows.

1 Soak hair thoroughly in warm water as you can't expect to dissolve sebum in cold water.

2 Use a small dollop of shampoo on short hair (a medium dollop on longer) by spreading it between your hands before stroking through hair to ensure an even spread.

3 Rinse your hair thoroughly as soap residue will contribute to the breakdown of the cuticle.

4 If your hair was greasy or very dirty, or the product didn't lather well the first time, shampoo again.

5 Rinse thoroughly again as it is very important to remove all soap and dirt residue.

6 Apply conditioner. If you hair is very long, dry, or chemically processed, you may need to apply conditioner the full length of the hair shaft. If normal, or greasy, condition only over the last few inches of 'old' hair.

## What's in a shampoo?

Most hair care experts now admit that all modern shampoos are so well formulated that you would be hard-pressed to find an unsatisfactory product. As a result, the only guideline we can offer is to buy according to price and/or convenience. You may prefer to buy an designer brand in a salon or an inexpensive one in a supermarket. Either way, your hair really won't know the difference.

Just as with skincare products, however, choosing the right type of formulation for your hair type is important. Shampoos, like facial products, tend to divide into those for oily, normal, dry and/or chemically treated hair and the difference between them lies chiefly in the detergents (yes, detergents, but not the dishwashing variety).

For example, shampoos for greasy hair often include anionic detergents such as the lauryl sulfates because they offer very efficient cleansing. They can be harsh on dry hair, though. Shampoos for normal and dry hair shampoos may include nonionic surfactants which cleanse gently and leave the hair feeling soft and manageable. Shampoos for damaged, permed and coloured hair often include cationic surfactants because although they don't cleanse or lather well, they make the hair soft and manageable.

## How sun damages hair

Just as in your skin, natural hair melanin provides extraordinarily efficient protection from the effects of UV radiation, not only for your hair, but more importantly, for your scalp. However, most of your hair melanin resides in the cortex where it is better poised to protect the living medulla (if there is one) leaving the outer cuticle less well defended. The layers of the cuticle are glued together by cysteine which makes up 20 per cent of each hair shaft. Cysteine is what makes your hair so fabulously tough.

However, the energy of UVA and B can break the disulphide bond causing the layers of cuticle to separate and curl away, allowing pigment deep within the cortex to leach out. What you

**beauty spot**

While your hair is wet it can be very vulnerable and rough handling can stretch and break it. Using a wide tooth comb, gently start combing bit by bit from the bottom upwards. Using silicone serums to detangle is voted by hairdressers and trichologists alike as your best bet for silky smooth hair.

see is shiny hair becoming dull and dark shades lightening. The damage is irreversible, until such time, of course, as your hair grows out and you cut off the damaged bits. However, you can prevent this happening. Sun filters can now be found in many hair products – from specialist sun hair ranges including sprays and waxes through to daily shampoos and conditioners. Using sunscreen protection on your hair is particularly important if it is already weakened by chemical treatments such as bleaching, colouring or perming, and also if your hair is long.

### Hair nourishment

Many shampoo advertisements promise extraordinary 'nourishing' properties of their formulations. There is little doubt that ingredients such as pro-vitamin B5 can, and do, penetrate the hair shaft through to the cortex but what good they do there is still open to debate. The best that can be hoped for is that they help fill in the gaps that daily wear-and-tear on the hair created and perhaps help fortify against future damage – at least until your next shampoo.

### The conditioning conundrum

It may seem somewhat perverse to wash your

*Modern silicone-based styling products have made post-wash tangles a thing of the past.*

hair religiously of its natural oils only to ply it with synthetic ones, but that in essence is what you are doing when you use conditioners. Conditioning agents, however, are better at smoothing and detangling hair than natural sebum. They are less heavy or greasy so feel better and allow the hair to shine, you can control where you put it (directly onto dry ends) and they smell better.

It's often claimed that you could forgo conditioner in favour of some vinegar or a squeeze of lemon juice in the final rinse. For healthy, oily hair this idea is sound; the acid would help remove any alkaline residue from the washing process which might leave the hair dull and unmanageable. If, therefore, you don't mind smelling of vinegar, it is an option. However, for those with normal or dry hair, specialist conditioners which include agents to help smooth together again the layers of the cuticle and seal in some water will result in a glossier finish and more pleasing feel to the hair.

Some of the older conditioners contained ingredients that could be quite heavy, particularly on fine hair. The latest conditioners are formulated with lightweight silicones which instantaneously smooth hair without weighing it down. As with shampoos, there is frankly little to choose between most of the well-known brands.

What your hair requires to be healthy and what you require of it style-wise are more often than not mutually exclusive. You may have thick, curly hair and detest its every wave. You may be naturally mousy but yearn to live life as a platinum blonde. If all we wanted was healthy hair, hair care problems wouldn't exist. But every time you brush it, handle it, blow it dry, perm it, colour it or vigorously rub it dry with a towel, you are doing damage.

If you cannot or will not live with the texture, or colour of hair you were born with, you will have to wash it more regularly, and generally condition it more assiduously, use sunscreens, and treat it more gently in an effort to persuade it to shine as it used to. But with a little mutual respect and some well-formulated hair care products, plus advice from your hairdresser, you and your hair should be able to compromise and live together in relative harmony.

## Hair Nutrients

Among the vitamins and minerals required for strong hair growth are:

- iron – found in meat, soya, yeast, wheat bran and spinach (although vegetable sources are not as easily absorbed)

- B-group vitamins – found in wheatgerm, nuts, eggs, soya and bananas

- amino acids such as cysteine and methionine, which are the building blocks for keratin and contain the sulphurs needed for strong intercellullar glue. They are found in nuts, seeds, eggs and meat

- zinc – found in cheese, brown rice, sardines, lentils and rye bread

- selenium – found in Cheddar cheese, shrimps, turnips and carrots.

Many vitamin and mineral supplements are available which promise to grow you better, stronger, fuller hair. You've probably heard it so many times that you're pulling your hair out with boredom, but you should get all the vitamins, minerals and trace elements your body needs to grow strong, full and shiny hair from your diet. However, it seems that most of us today don't eat

a well-balanced diet. Many of us restrict our diets to stay slim, and more of us are not active enough, so cannot eat enough to gain all the essential nutrients our bodies need for optimum health without putting on weight. Crash dieting, anorexia and bulimia, too, are widespread. As it is not a vital organ, nor even as crucial to our survival as skin, hair is often the first to suffer. Your first course of action in the pursuit of healthy hair should be to eat well. You should also eat regularly. Trichologist Philip Kingsley points out that after four hours your food intake has either been used or stored as fat.

**Iron** The missing dietary element which may be having the greatest impact on hair growth – or lack of it – is iron. Recent British government figures reveal that approximately 93 per cent of British women may be deficient in this mineral. This may be due to fewer, and later, pregnancies which mean that women are menstruating more often than they did a generation ago, and in part to the rise of vegetarianism.

Trichologist Dr Hugh Rushton PhD points out that it is possible for a blood test to reveal normal iron levels, and only a blood serum test will reveal the extent of a deficiency. Of the patients coming to him with hair loss problems, he discovered the majority of them to have low levels. Note to the vitamin junkie: despite selling his own iron and lysine (a protein co-factor for iron found only in meat supplement) he won't suggest patients take it unless tests prove they need it.

## Styling products

As styling products are going onto hair that is dead they can, therefore, do no harm. Most of them are designed to coat the hair shaft and make it more pliable to your requirements, helping to smooth and seal the cuticle. Those that contain sunscreens are doubly protective. Unfortunately when dirt sticks to them, they can dull your hair.

## Common hair problems
### Build-up

If you used a very 'conditioning' shampoo which didn't wash very well and then you puts lots of leave-in conditioner over it, followed by styling gels and mousses you would certainly suffer from a build-up of product on your hair. (There would also be a build-up of dirt as every passing particle would stick to your hair.) But you really don't need a specialist 'build-up clarifying shampoo' to divest you of it all. Most ordinary shampoos will wash it all away very efficiently, although you may have to shampoo twice.

### Split ends

Despite what the advertisements tell you, you probably realize that once the layers of keratinoyctes have parted company, they cannot be rejoined. You can, however, minimize the appearance of split ends and help smooth them down with a variety of conditioning and styling products: silicone serums, for instance, will both help glue and gloss over the cracks in your hair.

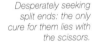

*Desperately seeking split ends: the only cure for them lies with the scissors.*

### Dandruff or flaky scalp

There are three possible causes of dandruff. It may simply be that you're not washing your hair often enough as skin cells over your scalp are constantly being shed, becoming glued in place by sebum and crumbling off. Wash your hair daily with a ordinary shampoo made for your hair type. If the problem hasn't cleared within a month you probably need to use an anti-dandruff shampoo. These type of shampoos contain agents to counteract the pitrosporan avali bacteria/yeast which lives naturally on the skin. It loves to feed off sebum, and so tends to reside in areas, and on people, where there's lots of it.

You will need to continue using an anti-dandruff shampoo to keep on top of the problem. If an anti-dandruff shampoo doesn't appear to be working, and your scalp is red and uncomfortable, you may have some sort of eczema or psoriatic condition and will need to consult a specialist dermatologist (see Chapter 5).

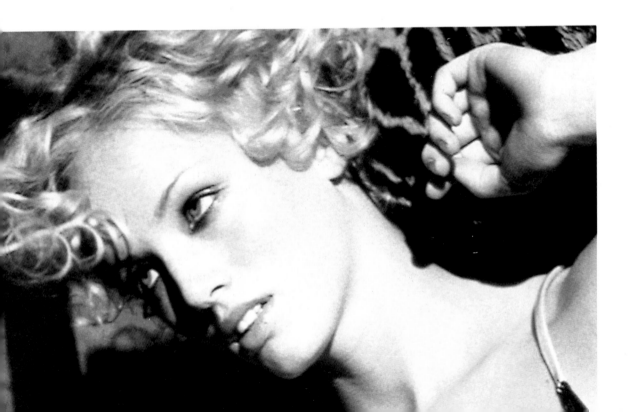

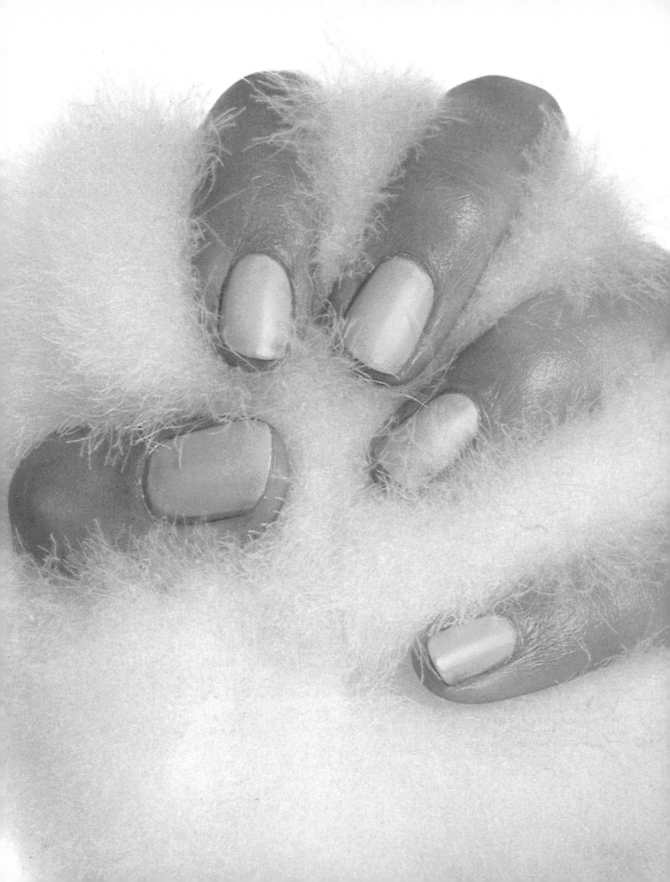

## Nails

**It is fairly obvious that your fingernails protect the ends of your fingers from damage. That nails are pretty useful tools is also clear. But of course, nails also play an important role in our appearance. Understanding how they grow and what nutrients they need to do so strongly will help you keep them in the style to which you wish to be accustomed.**

Nails, like your skin and your hair, are composed largely of keratin. The nail you see is manufactured in the nail bed which reaches almost as far back as the first joint of your finger. The pale sliver or half moon – the lunula – peeking from the base of your nail is where the keratinization which turns soft cells, into hard-as-nails ones occurs. In this, the lunula is like the epidermis while the nail itself is the equivalent of the stratum corneum. Like your skin, nail growth is continuous, but like your hair, the layers of keratinocytes are firmly bonded together for the life of the nail, or at least they should be...

### Eating for twenty

The very same nutrients that are essential for a healthy skin and hair are also needed for strong nails, albeit in slightly different concentrations. Your nails, for example, contain ten times as much calcium as your hair. Your nails require: B vitamins, essential fatty acids found in vegetable, cod liver and evening primrose oils; zinc; and calcium found in milk, cheese, eggs, yoghurt and green leafy vegetables.

But yet again, the best source of nutrition for nails is from your diet, not supplements. Unless you have been advised by a physician or qualified nutritionist you should not need to supplement your diet.

Many patients report that their beauty therapists and manicurists have often advised them to take gelatine to strengthen nails. There is, however, no clinical evidence that gelatine has any effect whatsoever on nail growth.

*Short and sweet: paints and polishes protect while they prettify.*

### beauty spot

● Your nails grow approximately 7 mm (1/8 in) per month.

● They grow faster during warm weather; pregnancy; after injury or illness; on your hands (as opposed to feet); and on your right hand (if you're right-handed – left if you're left-handed).

### Nail needs

What you know of your skin's needs is also true of nails. They need to be kept clean as infections of the nail area (bacterial and fungal) are relatively common, and they need to be kept well protected and hydrated.

To keep nails looking good:

● They need to be keep well hydrated: a normal healthy nail is about 16 per cent water. If the moisture levels drop below this the nail become brittle or prone to peeling.

● They need to be protected: the nails on the fingers of an 80-year-old are drier, more brittle and ridged and slower growing than those of a 17-year-old. It is assumed that nails are affected by ultraviolet radiation, but the extent to which changes are due to the natural ageing process or sun damage is not clear, not least because no one has yet conducted any such studies. While the jury is still out on whether nails need shielding from UV rays, what is certain is that they need to be protected from dryness – or more correctly, from drying out.

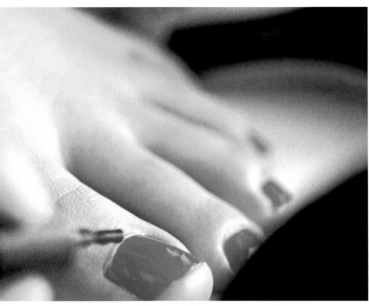

*Toenails grow less quickly than fingernails.*

## Protecting your nails

The moment of greatest damage in the life of your nail, it seems, is when it goes from wet to dry. Researchers at the University of Arkansas discovered that when nails get wet, the intercellular glue swells and softens and when they dry out again the glue cracks. This wet-to-dry process, of course, is precisely what most of us do with our nails at least several times a day.

## Sealing or moisturizing

Whatever your lifestyle, it's likely that for hygiene reasons that you will want to wash your hands regularly. In order to prevent your nails from drying out you should apply hand creams to them after you have washed them, remembering to rub well into the nail area. Many people have the idea that nail polish isn't 'good' for your nails, but in fact, it will protect and seal your nail from the water. It's also, therefore, a good idea to paint as much of the underneath of the nail as you can reach to extend the seal, and touch-up chipped polish as much as possible, as nail polish remover is extremely dehydrating.

## Polishes and paints

There are a wealth of different nail hardeners, polishes, enamels, and strengtheners available. From the dermatologist's point of view there is little to choose between them. Other than the formaldehyde in hardeners (see opposite) and acetone in removers, most of the other ingredients which go into nail products, such as polymers, acrylics, plasticizers, and resins, are relatively innocuous substances which are harmless to both the skin and nails. Also, nail moisturizers are now included in many ranges; if your nails are dry they could benefit from using them. The best idea would be to apply a moisturizer to your nails, wait until it has soaked in, then apply a moisturizing nail polish over the top.

Many different things can sap the strength from your nails:

**Detergents** Adding harsh detergents such as washing-up liquid to water is a virtual death sentence for nails. Although the intercellular glue is a worthy rival for the most super of superglues, repeated exposure to detergent-laden water will eventually erode it away. So wearing a pair of household rubber gloves to do washing up or hand washing is essential if you want to prevent damage to your nails and hands. Note: apply copious amounts of hand cream before putting on your rubber gloves as the heat inside them will help the cream's absorption rate.

**Injury** Most of the nail problems that occur, for example, hang nails, splits, ridges and white spots are caused not by dietary deficiency but through minor trauma to the developing nail – knocks, bangs, scrapes and even constant tapping away at a computer keyboard.

**Nail polish remover** The solvents needed to dissolve the nail enamels that we insist on being long-wearing and chip-proof are harsh. Try to limit their use to once a week or less. Some removers include moisturizing ingredients such as cetyl palmitate or castor oils in an effort to retard water evaporation. If you have a problem with nails that split or peel they are probably a worthwhile investment.

**Over-zealous manicurists** Many of the nail problems and infections that are seen in dermatologist's rooms are the result of poorly performed manicures. The cuticle, and the proximal nail fold (at the base of the nail) are often the object of vigorous 'softening', pushing and slicing during a manicure. But these areas serve a very important purpose – to keep bacteria and foreign objects out. You, or your manicurist, should not 'remove' the cuticle. You can very gently push the cuticles back when they are soft, no more. You can also gently rub them with some moisturizer – one that contains an alpha hydroxy acid, such as lactic or glycolic acid, glycerin, propylene glycol or urea, will help keep ragged cuticles at bay.

**Formaldehyde** This was once included in nail polishes and hardeners, but it is no longer used in concentrations about 5 per cent as it proved very good at inducing contact dermatitis in a large number of users.

## Common cosmetic nail disorders

There are many minor nail disorders that most of us will experience at some point in our lives, but generally there is a remedy or they resolve themselves in time.

### Grooves

**Cause** Horizontal grooves can be the result of injury, illness or drug treatment which temporarily arrests or alters the development of the nail within the matrix.

**Remedy** They may take three to five months, or up to two years to disappear completely, but they usually grow out. In the meantime you can render them less noticeable by using a buffing board or ridge filling nail polish.

### Ridges

**Cause** Some individuals nails are simply naturally more ridged than other, but more prominent ridging often develops with age.

**Remedy** Buffing to smooth them out and painting with ridge filler will help their appearance. (Occasionally the cause is pathological, i.e. due to disease such as rheumatoid arthritis, to growths in the nail fold area, or to psoriasis – see Chapter 6).

### Hangnails

**Cause** Most are the result of self-inflicted injury or excessive dryness which leads to the skin splitting.

**Remedy** You can snip the ends of the dead skin tag to avoid it splitting further (do not pull it as you don't know where it will end). To prevent further hang nails, don't pick at the cuticle area and keep hands well moisturized.

### White spots

**Cause** White spots or streaks are usually due to minor injury within the lunula in the nail which disrupts the keratinization process and prevents the cells from becoming translucent. The nail can also appear whitish if it separates from its bed due to injury or a condition such as psoriasis, or they can be the result of fungal infection.

**Remedy** If they are the result of damage, the spots will eventually grow out over the next few months and will require no treatment. If they are the result of fungal infection or psoriasis you should visit a dermatologist. (For details of other nail conditions see Chapter 6.)

**beauty spot**

Your fingernails actually heighten the degree of precision of the tip of your digit. A nail gives the soft tip of your finger something hard to press against when you are handling or picking up small objects.

# Q&A
## Questions & answers

**My grandmother and mother both have fantastic skin for their age, so will I too?**

Possibly, but not necessarily. Their fantastic skin is more than likely to be due to the fact that they spent more time out of the sun than in it. The rate at which your skin ages depends less on your genes and more on your daily sun protection. Your grandmother may not have sunbathed at all and may have worn hat and gloves until the 60s. In my clinic, many patients in their 40s and older express surprise and dismay that their skin doesn't look as great as their mother's, but these days we know why.

**I have wrinkle and age spots, but I never sunbathe so the sun can't be to blame.**

You don't have to have lived on the beach for your skin to be photo-damaged. Even minimal sun exposure is enough to contribute to photo-ageing. UVA, (the ray which weakens the skin's support network and is the main cause of wrinkling), is constant all year round, summer and winter, and unlike UVB is present virtually all day. For this reason it is recommended that you wear a SPF15 cream every day.

**My skin is really oily. Will it always be so?**

Oil production does fall off with age. If your skin has always been greasy this is a welcome by-product of the ageing process. In the meantime you can console yourself with the knowledge that your skin is less likely to age quite as quickly as your drier skinned counterpart – provided, of course, you stay out of the sun.

**I have been anorexic for the past seven years and my skin looks dreadful and my hair and nails are dry and brittle. Why is this?**

If you aren't eating properly your skin, hair and nails, as well as your general health will suffer. You probably lack the essential fatty acids required to make the lipids which keep your skin supple and well hydrated. You are probably also low on the vitamins and minerals which produce healthy epidermal and dermal cells, and aid their day-to-day maintenance. By eating a well-balanced diet you would probably notice a difference in your skin and hair within weeks. If you can't eat more, consider using a balanced multi-vitamin and mineral supplement.

## Will eating chocolate give me spots?

What you eat cannot make spots form from the inside out because, in fact, spots form from the outside in. If your skin pores get blocked with sebum (skin oil), salts from sweat, city grime, dust or make-up then the clogged pore may become infected and a spot may form. Acne is often the result of unbalanced hormones which cause an excessive build up of sebum. In such cases, eating well is important, and it is wise to avoid excessively fatty foods such as French fries in favour of a well-balanced diet with plenty of fresh fruit and vegetables. (For further information on acne and acne treatments, see Chapter 5).

## Are separate eye creams essential?

No, not necessarily. However, biopsies show that the skin around the eye is a third thinner than elsewhere which means that irritants can more readily penetrate and cause inflammation reactions. So when you use a specialist eye cream, it tends to contain fewer active, or potentially irritating agents, as well as hopefully having active ingredients to combat the dreaded crows' feet.

## Is it possible for my skin type to change?

Your skin could well be normal during the summer, but become dry during the winter when it is subjected to cold winds and the drying effects of central heating. Equally, your normal skin could become oily during the summer, especially if you live where humidity levels are high. Many people need to fine tune their skincare regime to the season, moisturizing more in winter and using more astringent cleansers in the summer.

## I live in a hard water area and my skin feels very dry. Would my skin benefit from installing a water softener?

While there have been no clinical studies carried out on the benefits or otherwise of soft water, it is safe to say that those with dry skin would benefit from washing in softer water. Hard water contains high levels of alkaline salts and the combination of alkaline soap and hard water can leave a drying residue on the skin. If you don't wish to install a water softener, try washing with pH balanced, non-soap cleansers.

## Is there any benefit in applying my skin cream with upward strokes?

Beauticians are often trained to apply creams this way and the leaflets which accompany skin creams often suggest it, but there is no scientific basis for the notion that upward strokes will improve sagging skin. Beauticians' strokes will normally stimulate the lymph system into draining away toxin-carrying fluids which can make the face puffy, in particular, around the eyes. They are also want to give you a relaxing experience. You can apply your cream in whichever direction you like as long as you do it gently and don't drag on the skin.

## Is wearing make-up everyday bad for my skin?

No, in fact, it may be good for it. Most foundations today are formulated to be non-comedogenic, that is, they won't clog the pores, and they contain ingredients designed to protect and moisturize your skin. Some of the best foundations actually contain sunscreens and antioxidants and are a useful addition to a daily sunscreening moisturizer.

### My oily skin won't wrinkle, will it?

It is true that fair, dry skin tends to wrinkle more, and earlier, than its tougher, oilier counterpart. Darker skin, which by definition is usually oilier, does have a greater degree of built-in protection in the form of melanin, but this dark pigment cannot be relied upon to protect the skin indefinitely. So, unfortunately, oily skin will also wrinkle if overexposed to the sun's ultraviolet rays. It will also show other sorts of ageing changes now associated with sun damage, which include sun spots, uneven pigmentation and sagging.

### Must I use an SPF15 every day – summer and winter?

The burning UVB ray is stronger during the summer months but the ageing UVA ray beats down with the same intensity all year round. Of course, whether you wear sunscreen all day, every day is up to you. If you don't your skin will age prematurely. If you do, you stand a better chance of retaining a firmer, wrinkle and age spot-free face for longer.

### Do skin creams work?

The answer, rather unhelpfully, depends on what you mean by 'work'. If you mean can moisturizers hydrate your skin, make it look brighter and feel more comfortable, then yes, they do work. But if you mean, can anti-ageing creams remove lines and wrinkles and shrink the sagging skin over the jawline to its teenage firmness, then no, they cannot. Cosmetic creams, by definition, can and should, deliver only minimal effects. Some cosmeceutical creams can produce more pronounced results (see above) but they must be prescribed and used under medical supervision.

### Moisturizer stings my face. Why?

You probably have sensitive skin which means that its outer layer lets in more than it should – and probably lets out more moisture than it should. You need to ensure that you cleanse it very, very gently. And don't apply anything which upsets it. Buy products from ranges designed for sensitive skin. Use SPF15 or higher moisturizing creams whenever possible. Such measures should help to shore up the skin's outer layer making it less sensitive in future.

### Could a new diet improve my skin?

If you diet lacks the nutrients your skin requires for healthy function, then yes. If however, you already eat a well-balanced diet then it's unlikely you will be able to improve on matters. Some animal studies suggest that a diet rich in antioxidants can help the skin defend itself against UV-attack but these studies have yet to be performed with humans.

### My skin looks better when I use a sunbed and worse when I don't

This is a common complaint of sunbed users. It is usually because the irregular pigmentation produced by the UV damage is masked by the tan itself. When your tan fades, the blotches become more evident.

If you suffer from a condition such as acne or psoriasis you may well be recommended by your dermatologist to use a sunbed. Ultraviolet light therapy has long been used to help clear the lesions of these skin diseases. However, there is a careful balance to be achieved between short-term gain and long-term damage to the skin. Trials in mid-1998 at the Hammersmith Hospital in London suggest that high frequency red light can not only help clear acne, but also won't damage the skin as ultraviolet light can.

## Is there any such thing as a safe tan?

No I'm afraid not. Melanin is produced in the skin in response to skin damage. Your DNA has to be under attack before it is produced so a tanned skin is, by definition, a damaged skin. The only really safe tan is a fake tan.

## I love to have a tan and am not prepared to give up sunbathing. However, I would like to go some way to minimizing long-term damage.

The most important thing is to ensure that you never, ever burn. Use as high an SPF as you can bear to. Keep in mind your skin type when buying and make sure it offers broad spectrum (UVA and B) protection. Remember too, that there is several hour delay before sunburn shows. Be prepared to build up your colour slowly and gradually.

## I like to use a sunbed before going away because I've been told having a tan is a protective measure against sunburn.

The melanin produced when the skin is exposed to natural sunlight does give some protection, but remember that it took damage to get it and even the darkest 'natural' tan of a white person amounts to a natural SPF of only about 5. Unfortunately, a sunbed tan is not as efficient as a natural one. For a start, the UVA rays of the sunbed do not cause the skin's stratum corneum to thicken which is an important defensive response. Also, the colour you get from UVA comes mainly from the bottom level of the epidermis, where UVA is more active, whereas the tan you get from UVB is evenly distributed throughout the epidermis.

## I was working in a bar in the Caribbean and often developed blistered, burnt hands. Why?

I think you might have used limes in some of the drinks you were serving. Lime juice contains plant chemicals called psoralens which cause the skin to become extraordinarily sensitive to effects of the sun.

## Can after-sun lotions save my skin and stop me from peeling?

They can certainly help to rehydrate your skin. They can even help to cool the burning sensation and make you feel more comfortable. Those with antioxidant vitamins may also help to inhibit some of the damaging effects of the free radicals which are rampaging through your skin. However, they cannot reverse damage done to your DNA, prevent your skin peeling, or halt the sun-accelerated ageing process.

## As my hair is starting to go grey its texture is changing from smooth and straight to wiry and wavy. Why, and what can I do about it?

The lack of pigment means that your hair doesn't have the same resistance to sunlight, it is not as full (the pigment itself made up about 8% of the volume of each shaft), and is no longer so able to hold moisture. Washing your hair frequently will help to put the moisture back in. Try using pH-balanced hair products including those that are specifically formulated for grey hair. You can also seal in as much water as possible with heavy-duty conditioners and intensive conditioning treatments. Use some sunscreens and sunscreening styling products, silicone serums to smooth its tendency to frizz, and try to avoid using heated styling devices.

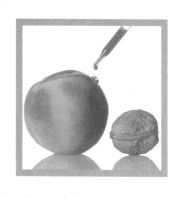
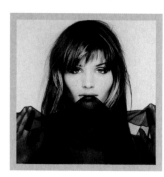
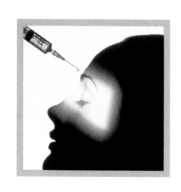

# skin problems solutions and anti-ageing treatments

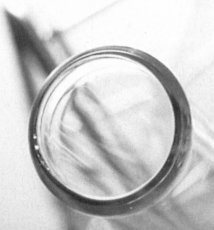

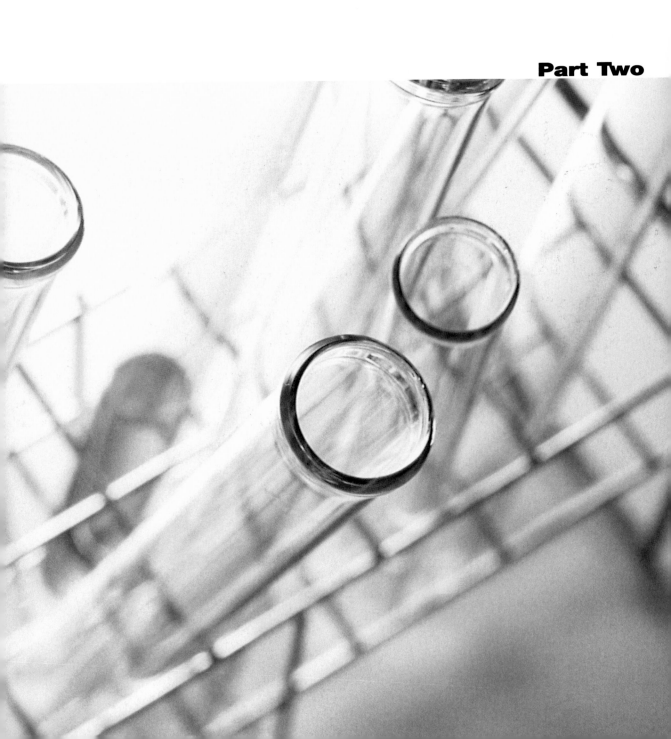

**Part Two**

# 5 THINGS THAT GO BUMP

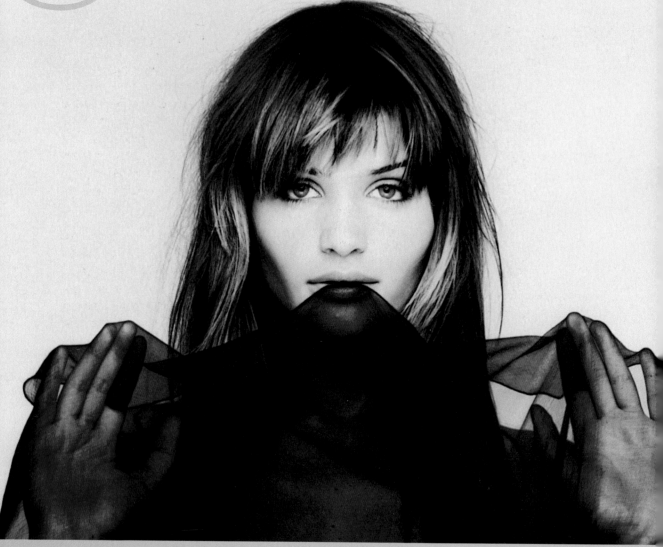

**Lumps, bumps, birthmarks, warts and moles – the list of skin problems is as long as it is colourful. And most of us have them, either for isolated bouts or prolonged periods. But thanks to radical new technology and drugs, few remain untreatable.**

# problems & solutions

With the exception of maligant melanoma – the extremely dangerous form of skin cancer which, if untreated, can spread and kill within years, few skin conditions or diseases are life-threatening. Many don't harm your health. But because they can affect your confidence by marring your appearance, they are often as, if not more, psychologically scarring as they are physically disfiguring. If you have, or develop, any sort of skin blemish – whether it be a thread vein you simply don't like the look of, or a ferocious and distressing psoriatic explosion, your first course of action should be to visit your doctor. If more specialized care is required, he or she is best equipped to refer you on. This is as important for so-called 'cosmetic' concerns as it is for other more medical problems.

Despite the fact that skin issues make up ten per cent of a doctor's cases, most still receive very little dermatological training. The core under-graduate medical curriculum may not even include dermatology. If your doctor does not seem willing or able to cope with whatever skin condition you present to him or her do not, therefore, be afraid to request that you be referred to a dermatology specialist.

## Spots, lumps and bumps

While your skin is usually admirably impervious to external events, it is often extraordinarily sensitive to your body's complex inner workings. From the hormonal upheaval that heralds the appearance of adolescent acne to the emotional stress that can bring you out in hives, many skin eruptions are the outward symptoms of inner turmoil.

### Acne

The appearance of spots – black, white or red (open comedones, closed comedone, papules and pustules) usually heralds the onset of puberty but contrary to popular opinion, acne does not just affect teenagers. It can persist into adulthood (see p. 78). While the condition can very often be a source of mirth and/or ridicule, spots can in fact be both physically and psychologically scarring. I (Dr Lowe), and many of my colleagues, are constantly frustrated by the length of time it has taken for sufferers to find help – very often five to ten years.

Many sufferers have been told for years: 'you'll grow out of it'. You may, but maybe not before the condition has left its mark. Acne can almost always be successfully treated, but the scars it leaves are less easily dealt with.

**Causes:** Acne occurs in those follicles that have a large sebaceous gland and a small, fine hair. At puberty there is a marked increase in the sebum production because of increased levels of the male sex hormone androgen (also present in women). This coupled with an abnormally fast turnover of cells lining the follicular canal leads to a blockage of the pore which can cause a relatively innocuous blackhead. If the natural bacteria (in particular *Proprionibacterium* acnes and *staphyloccoccus* epidermidis) then flourish in this hothouse atmosphere they can break down enough sebum into toxic material for white blood cells to be summoned, leading to inflammation and pus. It is possible for the infection to break through the follicle wall, which is when you get the more unslightly pustule-type spot, and possibly scarring.

Contrary to popular opinion, eating fatty foods or chocolate cannot 'give' you spots. Nevertheless, a healthy well-balanced diet with lots of fresh fruit and vegetables is without doubt better for the whole of you – your skin included.

**Treatment:** Wash your face at least two to three times a day to try and remove some of the sebum and excess skin cells which cause the blockage in the first place. For mild cases first try the many over-the-counter remedies available. Most today contain benzoyl peroxide or salicylic acid which aim to control bacteria and pore blocking respectively. (NB Abrasive scrubs are not generally recommended as they are often used too aggressively and can exacerbate your condition.) A dermatologist's first course of action in moderate acne will usually be to prescribe topical retinoids and perhaps antibiotics, the combined pore clearing and bacterial controlling effects of which can give impressive results. You may also have some of the lesions 'removed' in a controlled, sterile manner. (Note: never squeeze the spots at

home; doing so can rupture the follicular wall and increase the chance of scarring.)

Severe cases of acne, particularly those that feature many large, red, inflamed lesions, may require oral treatment with antibiotics and a tablet form of Retin-A (called Roaccutane or Accutane in the US) to reduce the activity of the sebaceous gland and reduce bacterial levels. However, both topical and oral vitamin A drugs and some antibiotics can make your skin sun sensitive so you will have to avoid the sun or wear oil-free (i.e. non-comedongenic) sunscreens.

There are other side-effects, too, which your dermatologist will discuss with you beforehand. Two of the main ones, however, are excessive skin dryness, and more dangerously, the risk of birth defects in a developing foetus.

**Adult acne:** An increasing number of adult women, many of whom never suffered from acne as teenagers, are now arriving in dermatologists' clinics with late-onset acne. The causes are varied but may include some or all of the following:

- Oral contraceptives which raise levels of progesterone.
- Stress – which increases androgen production (common in hard-working career women).
- The menopause – when androgen levels rise as oestrogen levels fall.
- Endrocine disorders – such as ovarian cysts or tumours.

The same treatment is used with late-onset acne.

A variety of creams and procedures can minimize the appearance of acne scars, but it's important to realize that none can make a deeply 'pockmarked' complexion baby-smooth again. For further details see Chapters 6, 7 and 8.

before and after treatment

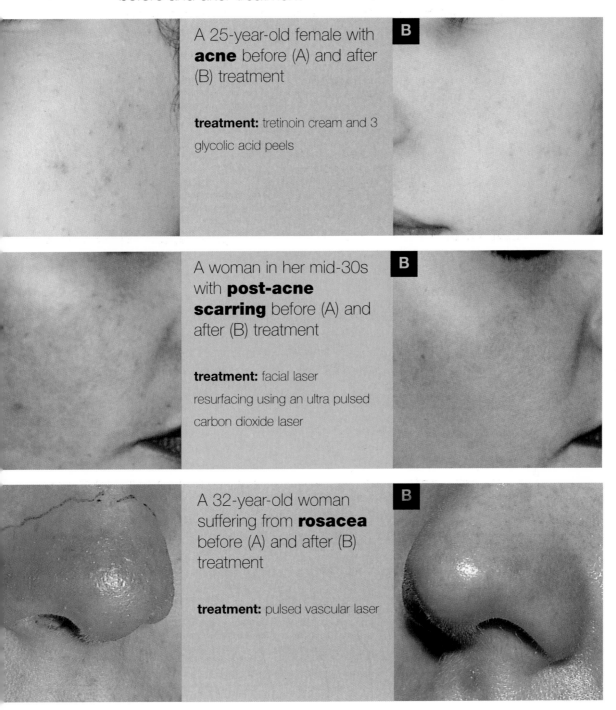

A 25-year-old female with **acne** before (A) and after (B) treatment

**treatment:** tretinoin cream and 3 glycolic acid peels

A woman in her mid-30s with **post-acne scarring** before (A) and after (B) treatment

**treatment:** facial laser resurfacing using an ultra pulsed carbon dioxide laser

A 32-year-old woman suffering from **rosacea** before (A) and after (B) treatment

**treatment:** pulsed vascular laser

## Rosacea

The condition is often incorrectly referred to as adult acne but, unlike acne, it features diffuse redness which resembles a fearsome flushing, generalized lumpiness, no blackheads or whiteheads but thin red lines where blood vessels enlarge (telangiectasia). In time, the nose can become swollen as well as red (particularly in men, for example, WC Fields).

Because it progresses gradually –sometimes flaring up, sometimes subsiding – many people delay seeking treatment.

**Causes:** What causes rosacea is unknown, although at various times theories about bacteria, mites, fungus and a malfunction of the skin's connective tissues have been put forward. The incidence of rosacea is higher amongst those with fair skins so it is thought their fine skin structure may make them more susceptible.

**Treatment:** Topical and oral antibiotics usually control the problem but if you have this condition you may have to continue taking medication for prolonged periods. Sometimes topical steroids are prescribed to help reduce inflammation in the short term. It is wise to avoid harsh cleansers and anything that can increase blood flow to the face such as alcohol (not a cause of the bulbous red nose as often thought, merely an aggravator), hot drinks, spicy foods and sun exposure.

## Warts

More of a cosmetic problem than a medical one as they can appear unsightly, these hard, crusty growths can, however, be painful if they are under pressure – such as under the fingernails or on the soles of feet (veruccas or 'planter's' warts).

**Causes:** They are caused by one or several of over 40 different types of the papilloma virus which invade epidermal cells and induce excessive growth and skin hardening.

**Treatment:** As well as the traditional, not always very helpful or often surprisingly painful remedies such as over-the-counter gels, surgical removal, electro-cautery and freezing with liquid nitrogen, lasers are now being used to destroy the enlarged blood vessels and cut off supply to the warts. Because they are expensive, not all hospitals or dermatologists have access to one, but some health authorities will authorize laser treatment at private clinics.

## Hives

Technically called urticaria (or as one of my (Dr Lowe's) patients calls it, 'hurty areas'), hives are red or white hard, raised wheals of localized swelling. They vary from insect-bite size to large, elaborate 'world map' type patterns and may last just a few hours or persist for up to six weeks. Most individual wheals, however, will fade without trace after 36 hours. Hives may feel slightly to incredibly itchy, or they may burn.

**Causes:** They are the result of an allergic-type reaction to anything from pressure (as in dermagraphism where just light scratching the skin can produce white wheals), to changes in temperature, emotional stress, food, medications or skin infections.

**Treatment:** Over-the-counter antihistamines will successfully control mild cases of hives, but more severe ones may benefit from prescription strength one, steroid injections or oral steroids.

**spot check**

If you have acne-prone skin you may also find your scalp gets scaly or dandruffy. Try using a specialist anti-dandruff shampoo such as Nizoral or Selsun and allow the suds to wash down over your face. The active anti-bacterial agents that treat your scalp will also benefit your complexion.

## Redness, rashes and sores

**There are many and varied names for conditions in which the skin becomes red, inflamed, scaly, itchy, blistered or sufficiently 'broken' to develop into sores: eczema (infantile, atopic or nummular), dermatitis (contact, seborrheic), and psoriasis (guttate, inverse and plaque). Although the different terms are widely used and accepted by the lay and medical communities alike, strictly speaking all are types of dermatitis, i.e. they feature inflammation of the dermal tissues.**

### Eczema

Eczema refers to any condition characterized by red, itchy, inflamed, scaly or even oozing crusty patches of skin. The term comes from the Greek *eczio*, meaning to 'boil out' which as anyone who has experienced eczema will know, is just what it feels as if the skin is doing. As mentioned above, strictly speaking, eczema is simply a generic term for a dermatitis-type condition. It tends to be reserved, however, for 'atopic' type conditions – meaning those that are not the result of contact with some allergen or irritant, but due to some sort of generalized, perhaps inherited, tendency to persistently irritated skin.

**Causes:** It is not known what causes eczema but it can be exacerbated by a variety of things (see list below).

**Treatment:** The first line of attack in atopic eczema is to avoid the following:

- Hot baths and heavy use of soaps.
- Tight, scratchy clothing.
- Anything which makes your skin hot and bothered, such as sunbathing or excessive sweat-inducing exercise.
- Scratching – it only inflames the already irritated skin.
- Stress – which can precipitate or aggravate an outbreak.

Depending on the severity of the condition your dermatologist may prescribe topical corticosteroids to reduce the inflammation and/or oral sedatives and antihistamines to calm both you and your skin. If the skin is broken, crusty and open antibiotics may be necessary to ward off infection.

### Dermatitis

This term is normally used for the sort of inflammation, redness, itching or broken skin that develops as a result of contact with a skin irritant – such as poison ivy, nickle, chemicals, cosmetic ingredients or detergents. Seborrheic dermatitis is used to describe the itchy, red, scaly skin condition that sometimes appears on the faces of those with very oily skin – usually around the creases of the nostrils.

**Causes:** Contact dermatitis is often mistaken for an allergic reaction but is more usually the result of contact with substances which irritate the skin, such as the harsh chemicals found in many household cleaners, garden fertilizers or certain plants, or some preservatives used in cosmetic creams. Seborrheic dermatitis is caused by an excess of sebum in which the natural skin yeasts flourish to a degree that your skin finds irritating. Because it is often accompanied by flaking, many people mistake dermatitis for dry skin and attempt to moisturize, which only aggravates the condition.

**Treatment:** With contact dermatitis prevention is better than treatment. Always wear gloves when working with harsh detergents, bleaches or anything you know your skin detests. If you suffer an inflammation, rinse the affected areas well in tepid water to remove the irritant and apply a rich, but bland, non-scented barrier type hand cream – lots of it. With seborrheic dermatitis, wash the affected area with an efficient non-soap cleanser, rinse well, and don't apply moisturizer. If the condition is widespread or unbearably itchy, a doctor can prescribe topical medications to control it.

## Psoriasis

If you develop raised red scaly or crusty patches over your knees, elbows, lower back or scalp, you probably have plaque psoriasis. Guttate psoriasis is characterized by smaller scaly spots all the over the body, while pustular psoriasis features large, weepy sores all over the body. In the UK about 1.5 million people suffer from psoriasis and in the US there are 5–6 million sufferers.

The name comes from the Greek for 'to itch' but for many people the itching is sufficiently low-grade for them not to even recognize the condition.

**Cause:** Frustratingly for physicians and patients the cause is of this particular ailment is completely unknown. What is clear is that the skin cell maturation process is abnormal with new cells taking a mere 3–4 days to rise from the basal layer instead of the normal 28–30 days. It is also known that stress – either emotional or physical (such as when you cut or sunburn your skin) – can spark a flare-up.

**Treatment:** While there is no cure for psoriasis, many new treatments are available. Most patients' skin improves by sunbathing. Your dermatologist will attempt to slow down the excessively rapid cell maturation process with a variety of substances, for example, topical steroids, salicylic acid, tar, anthralin or most recently vitamin D or A derivative preparations. With one of these treatments 80 per cent of patients can expect to gain at least 50 per cent improvement in their condition.

In severe cases, psoriasis might be treated with ultraviolet therapies (including PUVA – psoralen UVA) therapy, which must always be administered by a physician to maximize the effect while minimizing the damage. The most severe form of the condition, pustulur psoriasis is, thankfully, very rare. Because the sores are often open, painful and prone to infection, sufferers usually require hospitalization.

## Cold sores

About one third of the population carries the virus, which is far more than the number who have ever experienced a cold sore.

**Causes:** The herpes virus lurks in a nerve of your skin until the body's immune system is challenged elsewhere, when the virus leaps into activity. This can also occur after your first few days on holiday when sunlight depresses the immune system, or after a rejuvenating procedure such as a chemical peel or laser resurfacing.

**Treatment:** If used early enough, the anti-viral preparation Acyclovir (Zovirax) is helpful in preventing outbreaks of cold sores.

### spot check

While there remains no complete cure for psoriasis, sufferers should be encouraged to know that research continues apace. A currently experimental line of attack involves immune modulators that prevent the activation of the lymphocytes thought to be responsible for the abnormally fast cell turnover.

# Growing concerns – skin cancer

Despite what we now know about the damage that sun does to our skin, the incidence of skin cancer among sun-worshipping Western nations is rising at an alarming rate. In Britain the incidence has doubled in the last 20 years with 40,000 cases of skin cancer a year being reported (and possibly twice as many again going unreported). Of these 1,945 people will die, the majority of them (1,508) from malignant melanoma.

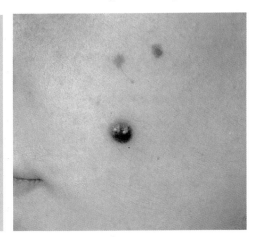

### Malignant melanoma (MM)

Learning how to recognize the signs of a potential dangerous melanoma is extremely important because they are the skin cancers which can metastasize, or spread, most rapidly and kill most quickly. As the name implies, melanomas are cancers of the pigment-producing cells, the melanocytes. If you already have lots of moles (40 or more), if anyone in your family has had MM, or if you have every experienced even one severe, blistered sunburn, you are at increased risk of developing MM.

You should watch out for moles with:

● An irregular shape.

● Uneven edges – whether raised and scalloped or flat and diffused.

● Uneven colour – moles which vary in shade from light tan to deep black or red with white streaks.

● Changes in size or shape, including if the mole is beginning to itch, crust or bleed. Any change, however minor, should be reported immediately to your doctor.

**Cause:** Although there is clear evidence for a link between the sun and other forms of skin cancer, we are not yet entirely sure how sun causes malignant melanoma. Certainly research has shown that even one severe sunburn can increase your risk of getting it, but because MM occurs in dark-skinned races and often in areas not exposed to sunlight (such as the soles of the feet and inside of the lip) it seems that other factors may be at play – heredity, for instance.

**Treatment:** A worrisome mole will usually be surgically removed, along with some of the surrounding tissue and sent to the laboratory to see whether the growth is cancerous or benign. If it is cancerous then further investigation will be needed. Treatment will include chemotherapy and/or radiotherapy, interferon drugs and possibly the new melanoma vaccines. Benign moles will need no further treatment but ideally should be checked, along with all others, by a dermatologist once a year.

### Non melanoma skin cancer (NMSC)

Basal cell and squamous cell carcinomas account for 90 per cent of all skin cancers. They are most commonly found in pale-skinned people, on the face, neck, ears and shoulders, on the heads of balding men and the lower legs of women. The mortality rate, however, is low (437 per 40,000 incidences in the UK) when compared to MM as NMSCs grow more slowly and are less likely to spread to the lymph nodes or other parts of the body.

Basal cell carcinomas are cancers of the cells of the lowest part of the epidermis. They appear as small, pale, shiny nodules, (sometimes with a concave centre) where basal cells have burst through to the surface without undergoing the usual keratinization process. They may sometimes bleed and/or become crusty. They grow very slowly over years, and if left untreated can eventually break open into ulcers but are unlikely to metasticize, or spread.

Squamous cell carcinomas are cancers of cells of the upper epidermis and are characterized by red to pinky scaly patches. Squamous tumours grow more rapidly and if untreated can grow into large raised tumours, sometimes with ulcerated centres. Unlike basal cell carcinomas, they can metastasize, but deaths from squamous cell cancer are rare. More often they are disfiguring as if not caught early enough large amounts of tissue will need to be removed.

**Causes:** There is a strong genetic link in the development of some basal cell carcinomas, but the sun is also an important factor in their development. The development of squamous cell carcinomas, on the other hand, is believed to be caused largely by the sun. The paler the skin and the greater the total sun exposure, then the higher the risk of developing them.

**Treatment:** Depending on the size and location of your lesion, your physician may choose surgical removal, curettage and electrosurgery, X-ray therapy, cyrosurgery (freezing with liquid nitrogen) or Mohs microscopic surgery. If caught in good time, the cure rate for basal and squamous cell growths is 95 per cent.

## Solar keratoses

If you have spent a lot of time sunbathing, or if you have type I or II skin and you notice a tiny, crusty growth, it may well be a solar keratosis.

**Cause:** They are the result of past UV-damage to the cells' DNA which renders their command centre incapable of correctly controlling cell growth and maturation. If left untreated, some of these small lesions could become squamous cell carcinomas.

**Treatment:** Although it may take years for such tiny growths to turn cancerous, it is generally wise to have them removed. Doing so rarely involves more than having a swab of liquid nitrogen held against them for a few seconds. If, for the general sake of your tired complexion, you choose to have a resurfacing procedure, even a very superficial one, you may find that this eliminates the solar keratosis.

Studies in Australia have shown that the use of Retin-A reduces the numbers of new solar keratoses as does the daily use of sunscreens.

### spot check

We are starting to see the benefits of 'safe sun' campaigns: the incidence of malignant melanoma is no longer climbing. For those who have already developed it the news is also good. At the John Wayne Cancer Clinic in San Diego scientists are working on a vaccine which may prevent the cancer from spreading. Trials of the vaccine are already underway.

## Coloured blobs, blotches and markings

**Just a few years ago the potential for treating a strawberry birthmark, a fine filigree of thread veins, the brown stain of melasma (mask of pregnancy) or the blue, green and black of an unwanted tattoo, was limited. Most of the options involved swapping mildly marring or deeply disfiguring pigmented lesions for colourless scars – a trade most patients were understandably unwilling to make. But the advent of the new pulsed lasers has changed all that.**

With the risk of scarring vastly reduced, if not removed (see p. 94), there are few such marks and blemishes that remain untreatable. There is palpable excitement amongst the dermatological fraternity, but of course, the real joy of lasers lies in seeing what they can do to clear the skins of those who appearance, and often lives, are blighted by birthmarks and other disfiguration.

### Birthmarks – red

The most common are: 1) port-wine stains which appear at birth and are flat red, pink or purplish. They can thicken and become lumpy with age and last throughout life; 2) macular stains which are faint, pink flat, perhaps streaky and usually small – sometimes called angel's kisses; 3) hemangiomas including 'strawberry' and 'cavernous'. The former are so-called because the colour and texture resembles the fruit, i.e. strong red and lumpy while the latter are purpley or bluish due to their depth within the skin. These often develop within the first few weeks of life and can grow rapidly but 80–90 per cent will have disappeared or flattened out by the age of ten.

**Causes:** Most vascular birthmarks are the result of deformities of the blood vessels or residual areas of the dense mass of blood vessel tissue that was present during the first month of embryonic life. The exact causes are not known but neither heredity nor activity during pregnancy is thought to affect their formation.

**Treatment:** The latest Flash Pump Dye lasers, can eradicate those birthmarks that time hasn't resolved or those that patients simply don't want to live with any more, even those impinging on the lip or eye area. A course of sessions is usually required for all but small lesions, with hemangiomas being the most complicated to treat. (For a more detailed description of the difference the latest lasers make, see below.)

### Birthmarks – brown

These include the café au lait – light 'coffee with milk' splodges and naevus of Ota – deep and dark-bluey black stains which take their name from the Japanese dermatologist who first described them.

**Cause:** Again, the cause is unknown, but it is reassuring for parents of a child born with a birthmark to know that there is no evidence that heredity or anything the mother did while pregnant is to blame.

**Treatment:** Café au lait birthmarks and naevus of Ota stains are treated with the Q-Switch Ruby laser, the beam of which is absorbed by the brown pigment produced by the melanocytes. Café au lait marks are usually fairly superficial, but treatment is only sometimes successful and the number of sessions varies from patient to patient. Naevus of Ota stains can run deep into the dermis but can be very successfully treated with ruby and alexandrite lasers, with a good chance of complete permanent clearance.

## before and after treatment

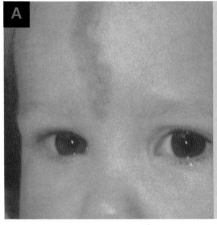

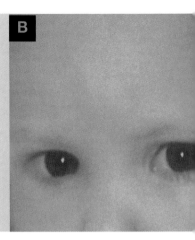

A nine-month-old child with a **'port wine' birthmark** before (A) and after (B) treatment

**treatment:** a pulsed vascular laser (see Chapter 8)

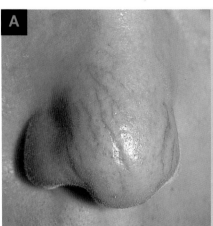

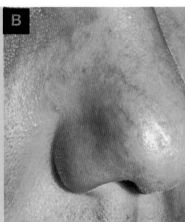

A 26-year-old man with **spider veins (telangiectasia)** before (A) and after (B) treatment

**treatment:** two treatments with a pulsed vascular laser

### Thread veins (telangiectasia)

Many people refer to these tiny, fine red traces that often appear on the cheeks or legs as 'broken' veins, but they are not broken so much as dilated.

**Causes:** There is no one certain cause but women are more likely to get them than men, heredity and skin type may play a role as may injury or long periods of standing or sitting. Anything which increases venous pressure may induce or exacerbate them and many women find they develop thread veins during pregnancy, so the role of hormones on circulation and skin

function is probably important. We also know that UV-damage weakens the dermal structures through which capillaries pass to the extent that the dermis no longer holds the walls of the capillaries firm and they collapse outwards.

**Treatment:** Despite the advances in lasers and the eagerness for many commercial clinics to use them, sclerotherapy remains my (Dr Lowe) preferred choice for the removal of thread veins, particularly in the case of upper leg veins. This involves injecting a small amount of concentrated saline solution or other irritating chemical into the

## before and after treatment

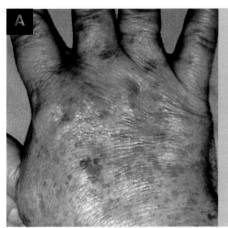

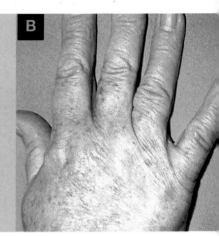

A 60-year-old woman with **sun spots or liver-age spots** (solar lentigo) before (A) and after (B) treatment

**treatment:** a Q-switched ruby laser

vein. This destroys the vessel wall shutting off blood supply. On the face and around the ankles, however, it is preferable to treat with the vascular lasers for reasons outlined in 'Risks', below.

**Risks:** As all facial veins run through the eyes and brain, it is highly inadvisable to use the sort of irritating sclerosing fluids which cause blood vessel walls to collapse; there have been cases of facial thread vein treatment causing blindness. In ankles, the nearby arteries can be affected causing ulceration.

Sclerotherapy also carries the risk of anaphylaxis, or total body shock due to an allergic type reaction to the injected fluid. For this reason, sclerotherapy should always be performed with a qualified physician on site who has recourse to the necessary medications for resuscitation. Other risks of sclerotherapy include bruising which may last for up to two years, blistering, the formation of a clot (not the sort that could move toward the heart with life-threatening consequences, but one which may nonetheless require surgical removal), or localized hives (see above). There is also the risk of the procedure not working – even in the best hands it can take two to three injections to clear a vein completely.

### Moles and age spots

The medical terms for these are pigmented naevi and solar lentigo respectively. Moles range in colour from light brown to almost black and can be completely flat or raised. They are rarely present at birth, but develop, and can grow or even disappear, albeit very slowly, with age. Solar lentigo (also known as senile freckles) are sometimes mistaken for freckles, but are usually larger and more irregular in shape, often appearing in later years on the face, chest and hands of those not previously prone to freckles.

**Causes:** Moles are clumps of coagulated melanin while solar lentigo are the result of sun damage which has thrown the melanocytes normal patterns of distribution into disarray.

**Treatment:** As long as biopsies have been taken and proven benign, bothersome moles can be removed using the Ruby laser. Solar lentigo are extremely common in people who have spent a great deal of time in the sun and usually appear in considerable numbers over the forehead, shoulders, chest and hands. Lightening agents can help to fade them, chemical peels will eradicate them, and they will also be some of the casulties in a full-face laser

before and after treatment: the effect of skin-lightening creams and peels for melasma

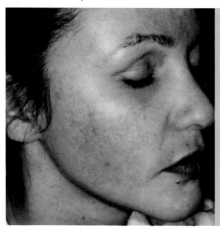

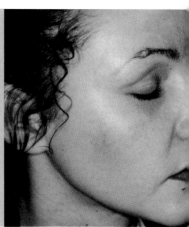

A 35-year-old woman with **facial pigmentation** (melasma) before (A) and after (B) treatment

**treatment:** lightening creams and glycolic acid peels (see chapter 8)

resurfacing to remove lines and wrinkles.

### Melasma (mask of pregnancy)

If you are in the second half of your pregnancy or on the Pill and notice brown 'stains' on your face or your chest you may have melasma. You are also more likely to suffer from melasma if you have quite dark skin (skin type 3 or above – see Chapter 1).

**Cause:** Some of the hormones which course through a woman's body when she is pregnant (or on the Pill) have the unwanted side-effect of increasing melanin production. Unable to cope uniformly with this increase, the skin dumps large amounts in certain areas. If you were to sunbathe when pregnant, though, you would get a double effect. The stains may fade with time, but rarely go back to normal. You cannot completely prevent melasma, but to help inhibit it you should use a SPF15–20 sunscreen at all times and try to stay out of the sun.

**Treatment:** Once your baby has been born, your dermatologist may suggest a course of topical creams including hydroquinone, koji acid and/or Retin-A. The same treatment would apply

to a person suffering from melasma while taking the Pill. It would also probably be suggested to come off the Pill. If these topicals do not have the desired effect, a course of superficial glycolic acid peels may be recommended (see case study, p.95). If small patches of resistant pigment remain they can be zapped with the Ruby laser.

### Dark eye circles

Some people with very dark skins – usually types IV and above – inherit a genetic tendancy to deep pigmentation around the eyes. This can make them look tired and one patient of mine (Dr Lowe's) even complained that people told him he looked sinister. In the past their only solution was to use camouflaging make-up – easier for a woman than a man. But we have recently discovered that lasers can bring dramatic improvement. The Ruby laser works best on those individuals with blackish-brown circles due to excess skin pigment – many of my patients are Asian or Middle Eastern – while the dye lasers tend to have a better effect on those whose circles are caused by very superficial blood vessels lending a red or even purplish tint to the skin.

*Right: Model perfect – just as magazines often retouch images by removing unwanted marks, so you too can now be retouched, for real, by the laser*

### Vitiligo

Vitiligo involves the total loss, usually in large irregular patches, of skin pigment. It affects 1 per cent of the population its most famous sufferer, (according to media reports), being Michael Jackson. Many patients with vitiligo are otherwise perfectly healthy, but thyroid disorders, pernicious anaemia, decreased adrenal gland function and alopecia areata all seem to increase the risk of developing it. About 20 per cent of sufferers report that other family members are affected. Vitiligo usually progresses in fits and starts with some patients experiencing bouts of skin bleaching followed by periods where no further pigment is lost.

**Causes:** Some believe it may be the result of abnormal nerve cells damaging the nearby melanocytes while other theories focus on an autoimmune reaction in which the body destroys its own pigment cells or an autotoxic one where the body poisons its pigment-producing cells.

**Treatment:** There is no cure but depending on the level of pigment loss your dermatologist may suggest de- or re-pigmentation. The former is usually reserved for patients with over 30 per cent of pigment loss in exposed areas and it involves taking oral medication to knock out all remaining skin pigment. Otherwise, we can try to persuade the melanocytes to produce pigment for the white patches by PUVA therapy (see p.82). It is very rare for a patient to completely regain normal colour but about 60 per cent of patients gain good improvement. Learning how to make use of camouflaging cosmetics can be as helpful as drug or ultraviolet therapies.

## Stretch marks and pregnancy

These consist of slightly depressed streaks a centimetres of two long which are initially red. They are usually found on the breasts, thighs or abdomen. Over time, the red fades to a silvery pale or even normal skin colour but the marks usually remain depressed.

**Causes:** Many women develop stretch marks during pregnancy but they can occur at any time of hormonal flux and/or weight gain – in adolescence, of course, the two often go together. Stretching the skin over a pregnant belly or around a pair of swelling thighs stresses the dermal collagen and elastin beyond its breaking point and separation of the fibre occurs resulting in small dermal scars.

But the physical stretching may only be half the problem. It is thought that the natural steroids present in the body during pregnancy, puberty or while on the Pill reduce collagen fibre formation and partially inhibit the function of fibroblasts. (Patients on topical cortisones have been known to spontaneously develop stretch marks.)

**Treatment:** Once your pregnancy, (or weight gain) is over, topical retinoids can produce some lessening of the appearance of stretch marks, and recently, some of the vascular lasers have been used to take out some of the redness in new stretch marks. There remains, however, no cure for them; nor can you prevent them. Despite what cosmetic companies or aromatherapists claim, there is absolutely no data to suggest that anything can prevent stretch marks. This is because the fibres which rip apart are located in the dermis which is literally and physically beyond the remit of a cosmetic preparation.

# Hair and nail disorders

While few of us are happy with the hair that we have – too fine, too thick or too straight – these minor complaints pale when compared to the misery of watching hair fall out suddenly from where you want to keep it as in alopecia or chronic telogen effluvium. However, these conditions normally resolve themselves, but sometimes drugs are used. The embarassment of growing excessive body hair in areas where you least want it, as in hirsutism, is easier to resolve with electrolysis or the laser. With many nerve endings surrounding nails, disorders that cause splitting or peeling can be painful, but can normally be resolved with topical treatments.

## Hair loss

It is perfectly normal to lose up to 100 hairs a day (see Chapter 4) or more if you gave birth a few months ago. But if you are concerned about excessive hair loss you should consult a dermatologist as there may be some underlying medical cause.

If you are otherwise healthy you may consult a hair and scalp specialist, known as trichologists. There are some highly respected members of this profession, but their reputation is often tainted by the number of cowboy trichology clinics which prey upon distraught patients by making promises they can't deliver on and charging exorbitant sums to boot.

**Androgenetic alopecia:** This accounts for up to 95 per cent of all hair loss. It is a wholly natural phenomenon suffered mostly by men, but to a degree by all adults (also by some primates).

**Cause:** Scalp hair is sensitive to the male sex hormone androgen which can cause a follicle to shrink and begin growing a short, fine vellus hair instead of a pigmented 'terminal' one. In women androgenetic hair loss tends to take the form of gradual thinning all over instead of the receding hair line or bald crown patterns of men.

**Treatment:** Approved for androgenetic hair loss, minoxidil (trade name Rogaine or Regaine) is available over-the-counter as a 2 per cent solution, on prescription at 5 per cent. It works by enlarging the shrinking follicle and prolonging the growing phase of each hair. But only about 20 per cent of users will get any really significant hair regrowth and it can be expensive and time-consuming to use. For men, the tablet finastyeride (Propecia) is also proving helpful.

**Other causes of hair loss:** Major trauma, surgery or illness can interrupt the normal hair growth cycles but there is often a delay of up to three months making it more difficult for sufferers to associate cause and effect. Abnormal thryroid gland function can also cause hair loss as can the use of drugs such as anticoagulants, anti-arthritis medications, antidepressants and some beta blockers. Crash dieting, too, may rob you of hair if your nutrition levels fall so low that there is simply not enough food for your body to devote to hair growth.

## Chronic telogen effluviu (CTE)

This condition describes any abnormality in the normal hair shedding phase, which can sometimes be suffered by perfectly healthy women. CTE also describes the sort of post-partum hair loss many women experience a few

# Chapter Five

Traction alopecia describes the sort of self-inflicted hair loss brought about by pulling hair out by the root – either through unconscious 'nervous tic' tugging or plaiting hair too tightly. It is particularly common amongst races and cultures where intricate hair weaving is prevalent. Doctors and dermatologists are often nervous about giving a traction alopecia diagnosis; patients are notoriously resistant to the idea that they may be to blame for their problem.

months after having given birth. Thanks to increased hormonal levels and blood circulation during pregnancy, nails become strong and grow quickly, hair is full and shiny, and the skin glows. But unfortunately while few notice any skin or nail problems after giving birth, many women complain of losing fistfuls of hair three to four months after their baby is born.

**Causes:** During pregnancy, the anogen, or growing phase of the hair cycle (see Chapter 4) is extended – so that each hair stays in your head for longer which is why your hair may feel and look fuller. But afterwards it's payback time and the delayed telogen, or resting phases, kick in, all at once, and many months worth of hair shedding occurs within a short space of time.

Recent research by Dr Hugh Rushton PhD suggests that an iron deficiency may be to blame when hair loss is suffered by otherwise perfectly healthy young women (see Chapter 4).

**Treatment:** No treatment is necessary as the problem will resolve itself over the next few months. During this time you should eat a well-balanced diet and ensure that you are getting enough iron (the best source is meat rather than dairy foods or vegetables), so that when the next anogen phase begins you are perfectly primed to grow optimum amounts of hair.

## Baldness

About 40% of all men between the ages of 18 and 40 show signs of baldness, rising to about 94% in men over 80 years old.

**Cause:** You have to inherit a predisposition to Male Pattern Baldness (MPB) before the other factors which cause it can come into play, namely the effect of androgen and age. Going bald does not mean you have an excess of androgen (despite the popular myth about bald men being more virile) simply that your hair follicles are more sensitive to it.

**Treatment:** Other than minoxidil and finastyeride (see p.91) there is nothing else proven to have any effect whatsoever on MPB. Many men, and those around them accept their hair loss gracefully, but some find it very distressing. However, there are new micrografting hair replacement techniques which offer really natural-looking alternatives to the old 'dolls' hair' punch grafts. The surgical technique involves transplanting miniscule slivers of skin containing two to three hairs at a time from the back of the hair to the bald patches. I (Dr Lowe) use the $CO_2$ laser to cut and 'shrink' the bald scalp –it is faster and involves less blood so the operator can see better and the patient heals faster.

## Alopecia

This condition involves sudden and complete hair loss, either in small round patches (areata), the whole head (totalis), or the whole body, eyelashes and vellus hairs included (universalis). It can be extremely distressing; many sufferers become depressed about their condition or stressed by the thought that it may get worse.

**Causes:** Again, the cause is completely unknown. Some believe it to be an autoimmune response where the body attacks its own follicles, others believe stress has a role to play but neither theory has yet been proved. Sometimes the condition lasts for only a few months, sometimes it comes and goes throughout a lifetime.

**Treatment:** Because we don't know why it

happens there is relatively little we can do to treat it. Much alopecia resolves itself naturally, but the earlier in life the loss is experienced and the larger the areas affected, the less the chance of recovery. Local steroids are sometimes injected or applied in an effort to calm any inflammatory response which may be inhibiting hair growth. Minoxidil, too, is often worth trying. It must be admitted, however, that spontaneous regrowth is the patient's best hope.

### Hirsutism

Excess body hair growth can be almost as embarassing as hair loss. Women do grow hair all over their bodies, just as do men; it's just that most of these hairs are vellus rather than strong, pigmented ones. What some women may regard as excessive body hair may in fact be completely normal for their skin type and origin – many Mediterranean and Middle Eastern people naturally have more body hair than some more northern people.

**Causes:** Certain diseases or drugs can induce the follicles growing vellus hairs to start producing thicker pigmented ones. These include any hormonal imbalance condition such as polycystic ovaries, malfunction of the adrenal glands, or reaction to certain blood pressure-lowering drugs (minoxidil was first prescribed for high blood pressure).

**Treatment:** Once the problem has been identified, it is sometimes possible to reverse the condition. In the meantime there are many hair removal techniques, the latest and most exciting of which involves some Ruby and Alexandrite lasers. They are primed to target the pigment in the follicle (which is why those with darker hair respond better), the intense beam vaporizes the hair and destroys the follicle but (if done correctly) leaves the surrounding tissues untouched. Although it is as yet very early days and laser device manufacturers are still tweaking the technology – adding refrigerated tips, for instance, to reduce the risk of thermal damage – it seems that the removal is long term, if not permanent.

**Risks:** Both electrolysis and laser removal carry the risk of scarring. Laser treatment can also result in the prolonged eradication of skin pigment surrounding the hair. This is more likely if you have dark skin and light hair. For this reason it is wise to choose a practitioner who is experienced with this very recent application for laser technology.

## Frail nails
### Nail psoriasis

If your nails grow very quickly but peel, split, part company from their bed, and are ridged and spotted with pits, you may be suffering from psoriasis of the nail.

**Cause:** like skin psoriasis, it is unknown.

**Treatment:** Topical or injected steroids, or the newer vitamin D derivative (calcipotriol) preparations or retinoids can help dampen the over-rapid cell turnover but can have a detrimental effect on the skin surrounding the nail.

### Grooves and ridges

Such imperfections are usually of cosmetic, rather than medical, concern.

**Causes:** Horizontal grooves can be the result of injury, illness or drug treatment which temporarily arrests or alters the development of the nail within the matrix. Vertical ridges can appear on nails in later years for no apparent reason.

**Treatment:** None is needed. It may take 3–5 months, or up to two years to disappear completely, but they usually grow out. No treatment is available for vertical ridges but you can render them less noticeable by using a buffing board or ridge-filling nail polish.

93

# Chapter Five

## Lasers – the new generation

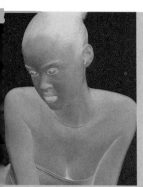

Even among traditionally conservative medics, the words 'revolutionary' and 'exciting' keep cropping up when talk turns to the latest lasers. But radical new laser technology is indeed changing the face of dermatological treatments. Previously untreatable disfigurements can now be eradicated with minimal risk of scarring.

Lasers have been around for over 30 years but much of the early enthusiasm for them waned when it transpired that the intense beams of light would not only obliterate offending blemishes of areas of skin, but transferred sufficient heat to the surrounding skin to cause thermal damage and scarring. Patients and dermatologists alike, were understandably reluctant to swap birthmarks or moles for scars.

Until ten years ago, things on the laser front had gone rather quiet. But behind the scenes, laser engineers had been beavering away in an effort to eliminate the problems of heat damage. In 1992 they developed a device which seemed to solve the problem: the pulsed laser. Instead of emitting a constant beam, these lasers 'pulsed' on and off in less than a thousandth of a second.

Because the laser's flash is so momentary, the heat the beam generates is too short-lived to be transmitted to the surrounding tissues, hence the potential for scarring is greatly reduced. Thanks, too, to advances in targeting technology, the new lasers are accurate to within a fraction of a millimetre, or to within one layer of skin cells, and so are safe for use even on delicate facial tissue such as that surrounding the eye.

Conditions and blemishes, such as deeply disfiguring birth marks can now be zapped from existence. There are also completely new applications for lasers. New types of lasers are now being used to sear wrinkles from crinkled complexions and assist in the micro-transplantation of hair grafts, rid you of warts, and remove the hairs from unwanted places.

There are currently about 50 different lasers in use, most of which emit differing lengths of light rays and come with a host of attachments and firing patterns At 10,600 nanometres, the $CO_2$ lasers are absorbed by the water content of cells instantly vaporizing it and indeed the entire cell. It is used for cutting and cauterizing, removing layers of sun-damaged skin and assist in hair transplantation techniques (see Chapter 8). The Erbium Yag is another type of water-vaporizing laser.

The vascular lasers emit wavelengths of between 532 and 600 nanometers which are absorbed by oxyhaemoglobin and so are used to eradicate lesions such as birthmarks and spider veins, while the Alexandrite and diode lasers are proving useful for hair removal and spider veins. Non-ablative lasers are being developed to try to tighten collagen for a 'face-lifting' effect. However, more research is needed to prove the long-term effects – both effectiveness and safety.

After five years of both clinical trial and practical use, the new ultra pulse lasers do indeed seem to have eliminated the problems of the old. Nevertheless, these are early days. Variations of this new technology are being launched every day and we are still learning about their possible applications. Despite potential for good, lasers are still destructive devices and should only be recommended for use by experienced doctors.

## Case study 1

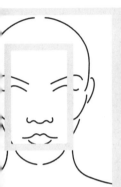

| | |
|---|---|
| Patient: | **Gail** |
| Age: | **In her late 30s** |
| Problem: | **Melasma** |
| Procedure: | **Lightening cream and a series of superficial glycolic acid peels** |
| Cost of treatment: | **£125/$205 per peel** |
| Result: | **Significant evening of pigmentation lasting months or years** |

### The dermatologist's story

Gail visited me as she was concerned about the brown patches on her face which had worsened

> Glycolic acid peels speed up cell turnover, eliminating more quickly the melanin-stained epidermis.

over the last five years. She is a skin type 3 and has been in the sun a lot. She was also pregnant nine years ago and more recently has been on the Pill. The brown patches were melasma and were the result of oestrogen and sun exposure.

I advised her to wear SPF15 at all times to stop further deterioration, and put her on a nightly regime of HQRA lightening cream, a 0.05 tretinoin (Retin-A), a 5 per cent hydroquinone and 0.05 desonide cream (my version of dermatologist Albert Kligman's Lightening Formula). I also advised a series of weekly 70–90 per cent glycolic acid peels which my aesthetician administered under my supervision. This had the effect of speeding up cell turnover and eliminating more quickly the melanin-stained

epidermal cells. After six weeks she has shown about a 75 per cent improvement.

### The patient's story

My skin is naturally quite dark and I tan easily. I have also travelled a lot and was on the Pill when I went to Cuba on holiday a couple of years ago. I had started to notice a brown line on my face, but when I returned from Cuba I was covered in brown stains and had racoon eyes. I tried all the sun spot remedies but none helped. Eventually, I was referred to Dr Lowe and was keen on laser treatment but he recommended a series of glycolic acid peels.

The acid stung a little, but I actually found the process quite relaxing. Afterwards I looked very healthy – really glowing – and went straight back to the office. I've had four peels and will probably have two more before we decide if I need any laser treatment. I am so pleased with the results – about a 75 per cent improvement. Regular make-up, instead of a very thick version, now covers the few noticeable areas left. The general texture of my skin is better too – it's so much brighter. In terms of the time and money I've spent so far it has been more than worth it.

## Case study 2

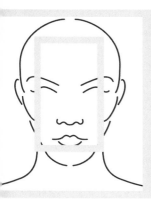

| | |
|---|---|
| Patient: | **Alison** |
| Age: | **27** |
| Problem: | **Persistent acne and acne scarring** |
| Proceedure: | **Topical treatment for acne, chemical peeling, subcision and laser resurfacing for scarring** |
| Cost of treatment: | **£3250/$5350** |
| Result: | **Complete clearance of acne and good improvement of scars** |

### The dermatologist's story

Alison consulted me because of her ongoing acne and also disfiguring scars from the severe acne she had as a teenager. I discussed with Alison treating her acne before the scars. I prescribed one tablet of oral Doxycycline (a tetracycline antibiotic) at night along with topical applications of a mild (0.025 per cent) tretinoin cream and azelaic acid cream in the morning. In addition, I advised four glycolic acid peels every two weeks to help speed the improvement.

After 8 weeks it was time to consider how to improve the scars. In the 'old' days I would have suggested dermabrasion but now I have considerable success with a combination of scar elevation (cutting under the scar with a microscopic blade to free the fibrous strands and inserting a dermal graft to raise the depression). Following this, Alison had an ultrapulse $CO_2$ laser resurfacing procedure to refine the skin surface and tighten the skin around the scars.

She is now using tretinoin cream twice a week as a 'maintenance' programme to prevent the acne returning. She also uses a non-comedogenic sunscreen each morning.

### The patient's story

The acne I had when I was younger had left me with scars, and coupled with the spots that I was still getting meant I was pretty embarrassed about my face and lacked confidence in my appearance.

I wanted to have the scars treated first, but Dr Lowe wanted to get rid of my spots first. To be honest, they were so mild compared with my teenage acne I didn't realize they could be cured. I had to take a tablet and use a face cream at night and to have some facial peels.

Finally my scars were treated. I had a sedative anaesthetic so I didn't know or feel anything of the grafting or the resurfacing. My face felt inflamed for a couple of hours afterwards, but the ice packs at the clinic and at home relieved the sensation. I'd taken a week off work so didn't have to see anyone at this stage. I went home with some sedative anti-histamines to take in case the itching irritated as the grafts healed, and by the third day I was glad to have them. What amazed me was how fast I healed.

It felt like a long-haul at the time, but I'm really glad I had the treatment. I never thought my skin could be so clear. The scars are still slightly visible, but they are not so deep grained.

## Case study 3

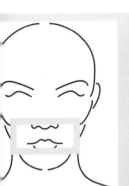

| Patient: | **Lara** |
|---|---|
| Age: | **29** |
| Problem: | **Dark hair on top lip** |
| Treatment: | **Hair removal using long-pulsed refrigerated-tip Ruby laser** |
| Cost of treatment: | **£150/$250 per session** |
| Result: | **Complete removal of hair persisting for over a year** |

### The dermatologist's story

Lara was an excellent candidate for laser hair removal as she has the ideal combination of deeply pigmented hair and relatively un-pigmented skin. This is because the laser beam targets brown pigment and in a person with darker skin and lighter hair the beam is less able to differentiate between the melanin in the skin and that in the hair. Consequently, there is a risk of inducing hypopigmentation or white patches. I used a medium 30 joules setting for Lara's colouring. For someone with even paler skin and darker hair I could set it at 40 joules while a patient with darker skin and lighter hair would require a setting of only 20 joules.

Hair grows in three cycles and we are able to treat only those hairs currently in anogen phase. I therefore advised Lara to return as soon as she noticed any new growth – which she did six weeks later. The third treatment was performed eight weeks later.

It is likely that she will remain 80 per cent hair-free for one to two years. After this time any regrowth normally requires only one further treatment.

### The patient's story

I'd always had more than a hint of a moustache. I used to bleach them but the blond hairs were almost as noticeable. When I became an actress I thought that for the sake of close-ups I really ought to get rid of the hair entirely. I signed up for a course of electroylsis because at the time it was the only option for permanent removal. However, it was taking months, I found the procedure surprisingly painful, instead of getting rid of the hair it often 'gave' me boils, and the cost was considerable – I was looking at about 30 sessions at just over £10/$16.50 a go. I was thrilled when I heard about the laser. It seemed the perfect solution and, as it turned out, I was a perfect candidate.

Instead of many sessions I had just three – each one taking just 10 minutes. It certainly wasn't 'pain-free'; I could feel each searing pin-prick but the anaesthetising cream I'd had applied an hour beforehand made it perfectly bearable. The least appetizing aspect of the whole process was the smell of singed hair. After each session there was a little telltale redness which lasted about two days but that was easily enough covered by some light make-up. Nine months later my lip is still completely hair free. And what's more a rogue freckle disappeared in the process.

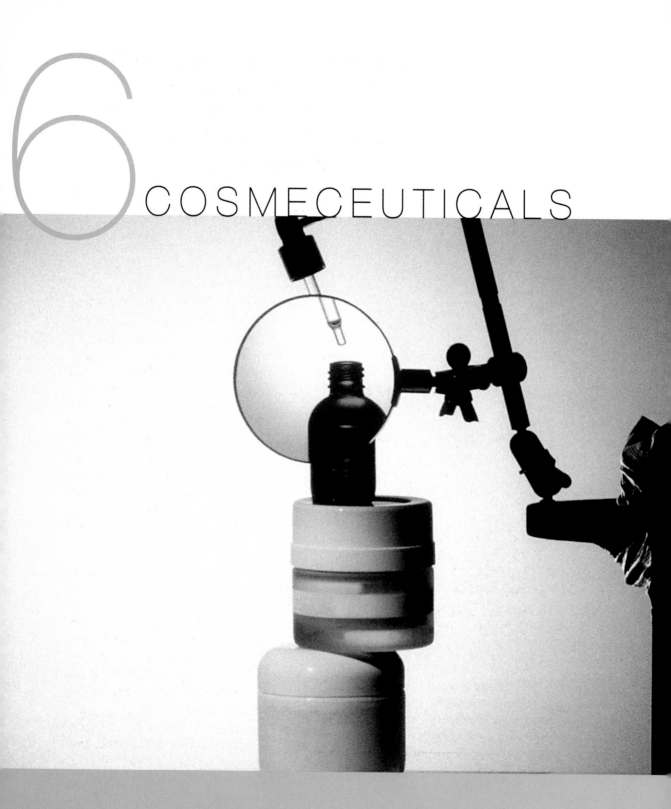

# 6 COSMECEUTICALS

**Not long ago if you had asked your doctor for a cream to remove wrinkles, he'd have assured you there was no such thing before sending you away for wasting his time, or, if you were lucky, with the name of a plastic surgeon. Not any more.**

# the term

cosmeceutical was coined just over a decade ago to describe a part-pharmaceutical, part-cosmetic type skin preparation that was administered not to treat disease, but to make aged, but otherwise perfectly healthy skin, look younger. Before the appearance of cosmeceuticals, dermatologists were skin

## Since the advent of cosmeceuticals, you can pick up a prescription for a gel which will iron out the creases of your crow's feet, a cream to brighten an ageing complexion, or an ointment that will fade your 'age' spots.

doctors treating disease, controlling disfiguring conditions and excising cancerous moles. Any attempts to smooth out wrinkles were left to cosmetic scientists while only the plastic surgeons could reasonably promise to shave away the years by tightening slack skin.

The sea change came in the mid 1980s. At the same time as the age-accelerating effects of UVA were being revealed, a highly respected US research dermatologist at the University of Philadelphia, Professor Albert Kligman, reported that patients to whom he prescribed a vitamin A derivative preparation for their acne came back to him not only free of spots, but without many wrinkles, too. It appeared that the drug, formulated to speed up cell renewal with the aim of clearing away dead skin cells before they could cause spots, was having the generally exceedingly welcome side effect of replacing enough dessicated epidermal cells with plump fresh ones to actually fill out wrinkles.

The potential of a true anti-ageing cream sparked a number of follow-up studies. Trials led by John Voorhees in Michigan fuelled enthusiasm. He noted that the cream helped to repair dermal tissue and generated new collagen, reduced the appearance of solar elastosis (the waxy pebbled look where damaged dermal elastin has bubbled to the surface) and of spider veins, and generally smoothed out skin roughness. In short there was an improvement in all the areas that differentiated old from youthful skin.

Once the news was out, scores of middle-aged women with sun-damaged skin flooded into dermatologists' rooms for treatment, while the physicians themselves proved more than willing to prescribe the vitamin-A derivative drug to the wrinkled as well as the spotty.

## The cosmeceutical – virtual reality

The term cosmeceutical is widely accepted and used by both physician and manufacturer to describe active ingredients that are designed to have a cosmetic effect, and usually includes retinoids, alpha hydroxy acids and some antioxidant vitamins. The law in most countries, however, has not yet caught up with the science. As it stands there are cosmetics, which are formulated to improve the appearance of skin, and there are drugs which treat disease by altering skin structure or function.

As a result, cosmeceuticals span the drug-cosmetic divide. Some, such as Retin-A, Retinova (Renova) and higher strength minoxidil are classified as drugs and remain available on prescription only while others, such as low-strength hydroquinoine and higher strength AHAs, are available as over-the-counter pharmaceuticals. Others such as lower strength AHAs, are treated simply as cosmetics .

particular, Scott and Yu noted that the acid dissolved the protein bond that kept dead skin cells attached beyond their useful life freeing the skin of its thick detritus. So if glycolic acid could clear thick scales of skin, imagine what could it do to brighten the skins of the merely mature?

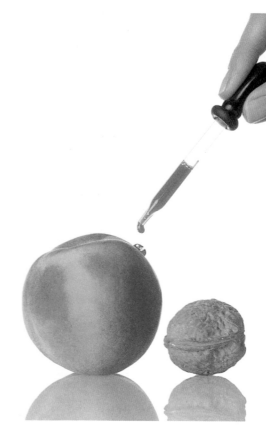

### Acid tests

A few years later in 1989, Dr Eugene van Scott and his partner Dr Ruey Yu were investigating possible remedies for the skin condition ichthyosis, an inherited disease, commonly known as fish scale disease, where extremely dry and thickened areas of dead skin cells build up to form cracked and crusty platelets. Working with alpha hydroxy acids, glycolic acid in

Similarly, dry skin of any age could be made to feel, look and be less dry in appearance when cleared of the dehydrated keratinocytes that characterize it. Also oily skin could be rendered less spotty by ensuring that dead cells were removed before they could block pores. Alpha hydroxy acids soon became hailed as a veritable panacea for all manner of skin ills. Unlike retinoic acid, the generic name for Retin-A, alpha hydroxy acids were not classified as drugs so were open to use (and abuse) by anyone who cared to concoct a face cream.

The third entry into the cosmeceutical circle, too, came as a result of research into disease control. At the University of Wisconsin, professor of preventive medicine Dr Lorraine Faxon Meisner and at Duke University, Dr Sheldon Pinnell were looking at the skin cancer preventing potential of vitamin C (ascorbic acid). An efficient free radical scavenger, ascorbic acid was applied to skin before, during and after UV-irradiation and seemed not only to neutralize free radicals before they could injure healthy skin cells, but also helped generate new healthy collagen (vitamin C is used by the fibroblasts to help produce collagen).

Having seen her colleagues Kligman and van Scott link up with pharmaceutical companies to manufacture and market the fruits of their research labours to an ageing audience, Faxon Meisner patented her vitamin C formula and began selling it under the Cellex-C banner.

Finally, three years ago, wrinkles were confirmed as not simply part of the natural ageing process, but as a treatable condition when a specific anti-ageing variation on the tretinoin theme was approved for prescription in both the US and Europe. Called Retinova (Renova in the US) it has a more emollient base to make it less drying and more 'cosmetically-acceptable' to mature skins.

The cosmeceutical is changing the face of skincare. Because of their medical parentage and the fact that they have been subjected to clinical trials, they benefit from a credibility never before awarded to the 'wonder' wrinkle creams offered by the cosmetics houses. Dermatologists who previously trained only in managing skin disease are now involved in cosmetic dermatology and focussing their attention on the reasons and remedies for skin ageing.

Previously incompatible, the cosmetic scientist and the dermatologist are now both working to formulate and prescribe or dispense the same compounds – albeit in different concentrations or slightly different molecular structures. And where once pharmaceutical companies made drugs and left the concoction of face creams to the cosmetics companies, now the two are also merging.

If your skin is sun-damaged, time-dulled or age-spotted, and you want to investigate what the upper tier of the new skincare system has to offer you, the following information will give you an idea of why and how you might use these preparations and what you might expect from them.

## Cosmetic cream or cosmeceutical?

The combined desire not to incur the wrath of the FDA (the US's ever vigilant Food and Drug Administration which rules on what cosmetic companies can and can't promise of their products) and not to scare away customers who have got used to extremely safe and pleasant-to-use products, means that cosmetics houses are generally restricting the concentration and activity levels of their products. This is as it should be. High concentrations can have side effects and only a trained medical diagnostician is equipped to predict how each individual's skin might react to a given compound.

As a potential cosmeceutical user, if you want a significant result it is best to get your cosmeceutical from a dermatologist. For a modest improvement you can buy over-the-counter preparations. (See also Chapter 2.)

## Retinoids

**The generic term retinoid is used to describe any of the vitamin A derivative compounds – from isotretinoin (Roaccutuane, Isotrex) used to treat acne, all trans retinoic acid (aka tretinoin, Retin-A, Retinova, Renova) prescribed for acne and smoothing wrinkles to retinyl palmitate, retinol or retinyl aldehyde (as found in cosmetic creams) for modest wrinkle smoothing.**

### Why you might use them

If you have spent a lot of time in the sun and are now showing the classic signs of the photo-damaged face – with lots of finely criss-crossing lines, areas of whitish pebbling (solar elastosis), cheeks that are traced with spider veins (telangiectasia) brown sun spots (solar lentigo), and a rough, dull, uneven or even yellowy skin tone – you are probably a good candidate for retinoid therapy. Studies have shown that tretinoin can help almost all these problems. It induces new blood vessel formation thus reducing spider veins and bringing a more youthful rosy glow to your complexion. It speeds up cell renewal and sloughs off dull, old skin cells so that it smoothes fine wrinkles and brightens the skin tone.

It also helps generate new collagen making the dermis plumper and firmer. As stated previously, photo-aged skin is distinct from naturally-aged skin in that its dermis is thinner while the epidermis is thicker. Tretinoin actually reverses this inverse relationship making your skin look and feel more like its naturally-aged self.

### Which retinoid to use?

For the treatment of photo-damaged skins I (Dr Lowe) prescribe either Retinova, a 0.05 per cent tretinoin formulation in a relatively greasy, emollient base or more usually my own formulation at 0.025 per cent. Retinova is good for a very dry skin, or for use on problematically dehydrated and sun-damaged skin on the arms and legs, but ironically, I often find that it's heavy formulation can cause spots in some people. My own formulation is in a light 'vanishing' cream and although lower in strength and so perhaps marginally slower to show the same improvement, it is usually better tolerated so you are less likely to have problems with retinoid dermatitis (see below).

### How to apply retinoids

Tretinoin is best used at night –for two reasons. Firstly, the agent itself is degraded by sunlight. Secondly, because it clears the stratum corneum of UV-blocking dead cells and brings plump, DNA-bearing ones closer to the surface, it increases your sensitivity to UV. During the day, therefore, you will need to use a minimum SPF15–20 sunscreen instead.

You should apply it to a clean face, preferably up to 30 minutes after washing so that your skin has had time to calm and reseal itself. If you are not already using a gentle rinse-off gel type cleanser you may be advised to change to one.

Your physician will tell you exactly how cream to use. You should not exceed this – more is not better, nor will give you faster results. More will simply irritate your skin more than is necessary.

### Risks and side effects

You may experience some light tingling to a stronger stinging sensation when you apply the

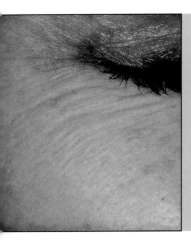
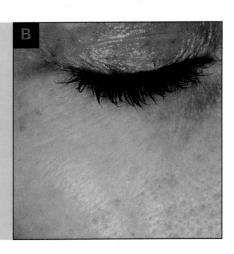

A 38-year-old woman with **sun damage and wrinkling** before (A) and after (B) treatment

**treatment:** tretinoin cream applied alternating nights with a 5 per cent glycolic acid eye cream

cream but this should last only a few seconds. Unless you have a very strong, insensitive skin, you will probably find that in the first few weeks of use your skin will display some signs of 'retinoid dermatitis', that is it becomes a little red, flaky and/or itchy. After two to six weeks, however, your skin should become resistant to the more irritant effects. While the dermatitis lasts, however, you may find it necessary to alter your skincare regime to include more gentle washes, blander moisturizers and richer, cream-type foundations. You should also exclude cleansing masks, toners and exfoliators.

If you apply the cream into the corners of your mouth you may find they become uncomfortable dry or even crack. This may also happen if you use too much of the preparation.

When taken orally, retinoids may produce foetal defects known as teratogenesis. There is no established link between the use of topical retinoids and foetal abnormalities, but for absolute safety it is wise to discontinue your treatment if you become pregnant. However, should you discover you are pregnant while on a topical retinoid there is no need to consider a termination; the very tiny amounts of the compound that penetrate the limited areas to which you are applying it are extremely unlikely to have any harmful effects.

## The results

It is likely to take four to six months before you start to see the benefits of your treatment after which time you can expect a 30–40 per cent improvement in wrinkles, particularly in the fine, crinkley variety such as those around the eye area. You should also see a reduction of uneven pigmentation, a clearer, smoother skin surface, and a generally brighter, rosier tone to you complexion. Deep lines, however, are rarely significantly helped, nor are expression lines as these are the result of profound dermal damage (see Chapter 7 for re-surfacing options).

When Retin-A was first prescribed for anti-ageing reasons it was thought that the stronger the preparation and the more irritation the patient could tolerate, the better the results would be. We now know that equally impressive results can be achieved simply by using a lower concentration preparation over a longer time.

## Alpha hydroxy acids

**This group of organic chemicals includes glycolic, lactic, citric, pyruvic, malic and tartaric acids. Often called fruit acids because of their origins (glycolic comes from sugar cane, lactic from fermented milk, citric from citrus fruits, pyruvic from papaya, malic from apples and tartaric from fermented grapes) they are now more usually synthesized for cosmetic use.**

We like to think of alpha hydroxy acids as representing exciting new skin smoothing solutions but they are actually the oldest cosmeceuticals – by many centuries. When Cleopatra bathed in ass's milk she was treating her skin with the surface refining and hydrating qualities of lactic acid. And when women rubbed the residue from the bottom of the wine barrel into the faces they were benefiting from the smoothing effects of tartaric acid.

AHAs refine the skin's outer layer by dissolving the protein bond that keep the flattened, anucleic keratinocytes attached to the stratum corneum. Rid of its scaly build up, the skin feels smoother and looks brighter too.

The work that Van Scott and Ruey did with AHAs also showed that they increase mucopolysaccharide synthesis (the process that helps skin retain higher moisture levels). They also act on the deeper dermal layers by increasing collagen synthesis and so potentially making the dermis fuller and firmer. Further studies by Nicholas Perricone published in the Journal of Geriatric Dermatology (1:101, 1993) also suggest that AHAs have antioxidant effects and so can be helpful in inhibiting the effects of sun or smoke generated free radicals.

Because they are not classified as drugs, AHAs are today incorporated into all manner of skin products – from washes and exfoliators to day creams and masks. Cosmetics creams tend to incorporate 1–8 per cent AHAs, specialist salon ranges up to 15 per cent and physician dispensed ranges anywhere up to about 20 per cent. Concentrations of 30–90 per cent are also used to perform peels, see Chapter 8).

## Why you might use them

The applications for AHAs are wide and varied. If your skin is prone to spots, an AHA preparation can help clear the pore-plugging cells that cause them. If your skin is rough and dry, AHAs can smooth it and make it better able to hold moisture. If your complexion has dulled with age, AHAs can brighten it. They may also help to lighten dark spots and melasma maybe by increasing cell turnover beyond the pigment-injecting capacity of the melanocytes.

## Which AHAs to use?

There are many cosmetic AHA preparations now available over the counter, for example Estée Lauder's Fruition, La Prairie Age Management and L'Oreal's Excell range, each boasting its own superior cocktail of different acids, usually at 8% or much less. The companies tend to forgo more spectacular results in favour of producing products which are completely safe and pleasant to use meaning you can probably buy and use them with impunity.

Because it is the most widely studied and believed to be the most effective, most of the dermatologist- or specialist salon-dispensed preparations (MD Formulations, MD Forté,

Murad, Neostrata to name a few) are based on 10–20 per cent glycolic acid. Glycolic acid's efficacy is probably due to its size – it is the smallest AHA molecule (with only two carbon atoms to pyruvic's eight) and so can penetrate further into the skin. It gives more rapid and marked results but can sting more on application – one of the reasons cosmetic companies are reluctant to use it.

AHA body products can be extremely useful for the care and control of dry body skin. A well-formulated product will make rough knees and elbows silky smooth almost instantly.

### How to apply AHAs

If you're using a cosmetic AHA you could probably apply it morning and night with no adverse effects. A physician-only type AHA will probably be recommended for use at night only, again on a clean face.

If, however, you are using both Retin-A and an AHA formulation you may use the Retin-A at night and AHAs in the morning. This allows time for their different actions to take place (see below). Using an AHA in the morning also helps to put a useful barrier between your naturally acidic skin and often alkaline make-up products which can upset the skin's normal function. If you are advised to use both it is best to use them on alternate nights – one to refine and to increase the penetration of the other.

**spot check**

A paper by Albert Kligman published in the Journal of Geriatric Dermatology 1:179, 1993 suggests the results from the combined use of a retinoid and an AHA may be greater than the sum of the parts. This may be because the barrier refining effects of alpha hydroxy acids improve the skin's tolerance to tretinoin allowing the use of a higher concentration.

### Risks and side effects

Most AHAs will sting or at least tingle slightly on application but the feeling should subside within 30 seconds. The degree of reaction will depend on the acid concentration and your particular skin type. Some people notice very little or nothing at all.

Because the acid clears and thins the stratum corneum which makes up part of your skin's natural sun shield, it is wise to use a daily sunscreen of at least SPF15 when using AHAs.

If you have sensitive skin you may find AHAs very irritating; the stinging may be persistent, or even intolerable and your skin can become red and inflamed. If this is the case you should stop using them. It's possible that your stratum corneum is too broken down to cope with them. However, by initiating a sensitive skincare regime (see Chapter 2) your skin might tolerate them better in the future.

Because you can buy so many different sorts of AHA products there are worries among some skin specialists that their overuse could denude your stratum corneum of too many cells leaving it prone to irritation. However, I (Dr Lowe) haven't yet seen patients with any AHA-induced problems and complaints to the cosmetics ruling bodies about them are notably few and far between.

### Results

One of the gratifying things about AHAs is that their effects are almost instantaneous. Your skin should feel smoother within days. Your complexion should look brighter and within weeks you will probably notice that your previously dry skin needs less moisturizer to remain feeling comfortable and looking plump and moist, or that your oily skin develops fewer spots. (See also AHA peels Chapter 7.)

## Beta hydroxy acids

**The only BHA in use in modern cosmetic dermatology is salicylic acid. Originally extracted from willow bark (the source of aspirin), it was been incorporated into pharmaceutical and cosmetic skincare products for over 100 years.**

The difference between AHA and BHAs lies in the position of the hydroxy group – at the alpha position of the molecule in the former and the beta position in the latter. In other words, the difference is too minimal for the average user to bother about. Just like AHAs, salicylic acid is very effective at dissolving superfluous cells of the stratum corneum but unlike AHAs, it also has an anti-inflammatory effect.

**spot check**

Salicylic acid is the active ingredient, if not the cornerstone, of the Clinique range of skin products. It can also be found in over-the-counter, anti-spot remedies.

### Why you might use BHAs

If your skin is prone to spots rather than wrinkles, (or is both spotty and wrinkled!) your physician may treat your skin with salicylic acid. The combined effects of unblocking pores and the anti-inflammatory action will help tp prevent future spots, clear existing blackheads and calm inflamed spos. Salicylic acd is best suited, however, to mild acne as its action is limited. (For modeate or severe acne, retinoid therapy is more effective.) The advantage, however, is that its side effects, too, are limited, if not neglible.

### Which BHA to use?

Salicylic acid is the only BHA in current cosmetic dermatologic use. It is available in some cosmetic creams, such as Clinique's Turnaround and Almay's Time Off creams and in dermatological preparations such as those in the Medicis range which is used for peels. Your physician will decide whether you will benefit more from an AHA or BHA or a combination.

### How to apply BHAs

Salicylic acid is often incorporated into toner-type lotions, exfoliators, washes for acne-prone skin or leave-on spot remedies. Creams are best used at night when the skin is free of make-up but can be used during the day under a sunscreen, if desired.

### Risks and side effects

Like AHA preparations, salicylic acid can sting on application. Similarly, its overuse could theoretically make your skin more sensitive to other preparations. You can limit the stinging by ensuring your cleanser is a gentle one, leaving 10 minutes to half an hour between washing your face and applying the cream, or applying it every second night only.

### Results

You should notice a marked smoothing of your skin's surface, and also a reduced tendency to develop any spots.

# Ascorbates

**Ascorbic acid, or vitamin C, was first proposed as an anti-ageing treatment to inhibit age-related and cancerous changes caused by free radicals. As vitamin C also aids collagen production, it was thought that topical applications might help plump up a deflating dermis.**

Early studies using vitamin C at Duke University, North Carolina and the University of Wisconsin, by Dr Sheldon Pinnell and Dr Lorraine Faxon Meisner respectively, showed promise but later studies have failed to duplicate the results. There is little doubt that vitamin C is an efficient free radical scavenger and can probably help defend and repair some degree of photo damage. There is, as yet, however, precious little data to support the use of ascorbic acid for new collagen formation.

I (Dr Lowe) do use and dispense vitamin C-containing preparations (Cellex-C is Dr Faxon Meisner's own patented formulation) largely for their free radical quenching capacity and in the hope that further studies may yet show benefits to collagen formation.

## Why you might use them

Like many dermatologic and plastic surgeons I often suggest the use of ascorbates to patients about to undergo a surgical or resurfacing procedure. The thinking is that a reservoir of vitamin C will be built up to both help neutralize the free radicals created by the injury (any damage creates free radicals) and supply the catalysts needed by the fibroblasts for new collagen production and tissue healing.

## Which ascorbates to use?

The two main proponents in the vitamin-C story now both sell their formulations (Faxon Meisner's is Cellex-C and Pinnell's forms part of the Skinceuticals range, both available without prescription from dermatologists or specialist salons). Both have vitamin C available in cream and serum form. I prefer the creams because it

is easier to control the dose. High concentrations of vitamin C can be irritating to skin and it's easier to apply more serum than is necessary.

Although vitamin C is a very tricky molecule to stabilize, many cosmetic companies now claim to have done so and are marketing vitamin-C containing creams. If this is the case, they may well be useful as day creams as an adjunct to sunscreens to help defend against sun and pollution-induced free radical damage.

## How to apply ascorbates

Stroke onto clean face at night in small amounts. If it stings wait longer after washing. The skin's sebum helps to slow down the rate of penetration. Some of my colleagues also suggest that the committed sun worshippers apply them in morning under their sunscreen for free radical quenching reasons.

## Risks and side effects

The only reported unwelcome effects of ascorbates are stinging on application and some redness and irritation. These can be avoided by using less of the product and/or applying it on alternate nights only.

## Results

Company literature for the two preparations currently available, discuss firmer, younger-looking skin but there is little independent data to support this. At the moment, results of the French government SU.VI.MAX study suggest however, that the preventive rather than reparative effects of antioxidant vitamins such as vitamin C may yet prove to be of greatest long-term benefit to our skin.

# Chapter six

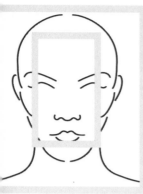

## Case study 1

| | |
|---|---|
| Patient: | **Fiona** |
| Age: | **33** |
| Problem: | **Oily skin, prone to spots** |
| Procedure: | **Topical AHAs** |
| Cost of treatment: | **AHA creams: £50/$80; glycolic acid peels: £125/$200 each** |
| Result: | **Clearance of spots, general improvement of complexion** |

### The dermatologist's story

Fiona had a history of acne and was still suffering from some open and close comedones (white- and blackheads). She was also concerned about the overall tone of her skin – she

> ## She was concerned about the overall tone of her skin – she complained of open pores, greasiness and dullness

complained of open pores, greasiness and dullness. I advised her to step up her cleansing regime and to use a cleanser formulated specifically for oily skin morning and night. I also prescribed a 0.025 tretinoin cream and a mild 15 per cent glycolic acid-containing cream for use on alternative nights. Before this treatment she had a series of glycolic acid peels (50 per cent for two minutes, increasing to 70 per cent for four minutes). After six peels over six weeks her skin had significantly improved, and she is now continuing with the cream treatments mentioned and having a monthly 50 per cent glycolic acid peel. She may continue this regime indefinitely.

### The patient's story

I went to see Dr Lowe because I was unhappy with the general texture of my skin. I had suffered from acne as a teenager and was treated with oral antibiotics, but was still getting a few spots. Also my complexion was generally dull and tired looking and I had visible open pores and some fine lines. He suggested a series of peels to kick start the process before putting me on to nightly applications of glycolic acid cream.

The cream can sting a little on application but only for a few seconds. I actually quite liked the feeling. I took it as a sign that something was happening.

The treatment has certainly done what I was told it would do. My skin is smoother and much brighter looking and if I look closely my facial lines seem softer. Although my forehead is still a bit shiny, the rest of my faces if much less oily. The most marked difference is that I don't seem to get spots nearly as often. Things are definitely improved – and it was very easy.

## Case study 2

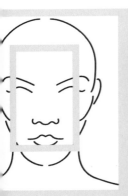

| | |
|---|---|
| Patient: | **Joyce** |
| Age: | **54** |
| Problem: | **Sun damage and wrinkling** |
| Procedure: | **Tretinoin cream treatment** |
| Cost of treatment: | **£15/$40** |
| Result: | **Significant improvement in skin smoothness, moderate improvement in wrinkles** |

### The dermatologist's story

Joyce had been in the sun a great deal, and although she is skin type 3 and tans easily, her skin nevertheless showed some of the classic signs of UV-induced ageing which included uneven pigmentation, a roughened, thickened epidermis and a generally dull complexion.

I prescribed a 0.025 per cent concentration to apply nightly, because although her skin would probably tolerate a higher strength neither she nor I wanted to risk retinoid dermatitis. Besides, we now know that equally good results can be achieved using a lower concentration formula over a longer period of time. She left with an instruction leaflet which told her when and how much to apply and she was also told that if she developed excessive redness or flaking, she should apply the cream every other night and call the clinic if she had any queries. An appointment was made for a month later to monitor her progress. She experienced no problems and after four months she showed a 30 per cent improvement in the fine lines around her eyes and mouth, and a 70 per cent improvement in skin smoothness and uniformity of pigmentation. She does not like having to wear sunscreens on a daily basis, but is happy with the result.

### The patient's story

I've always loved to sunbathe, so when I read about a cream that could help reverse some of the damage I'd done I leapt at the chance. I always knew I would never be brave enough to consider surgery, but reckoned I could cope with some cream. However, I didn't want to get retinoid dermatitis so was glad of the option of the slower-but-surer route with the lower-strength cream, but did have to restrain myself from using too much. I'd been told that it would take three to four months to see a difference in my skin, but I noticed something happening after just a couple of weeks. Already my skin seemed much smoother and brighter, and where it had been a bit sallow I had a lovely pink glow.

Over the first few weeks my skin was a little flaky, but I didn't mind as I could rub the patches away in the morning and it was a reassuring sign of progress. After four months the general texture and tone of my skin was as I had been told to expect – fresher, firmer and brighter. I can barely find the age spots I had on my cheeks and, although my deep lines are still there, the fine lines are a great deal softer. I'm very satisfied with the results. The thing I find most tricky is having to wear sunscreen all the time. I really miss being able to put my face in the sun.

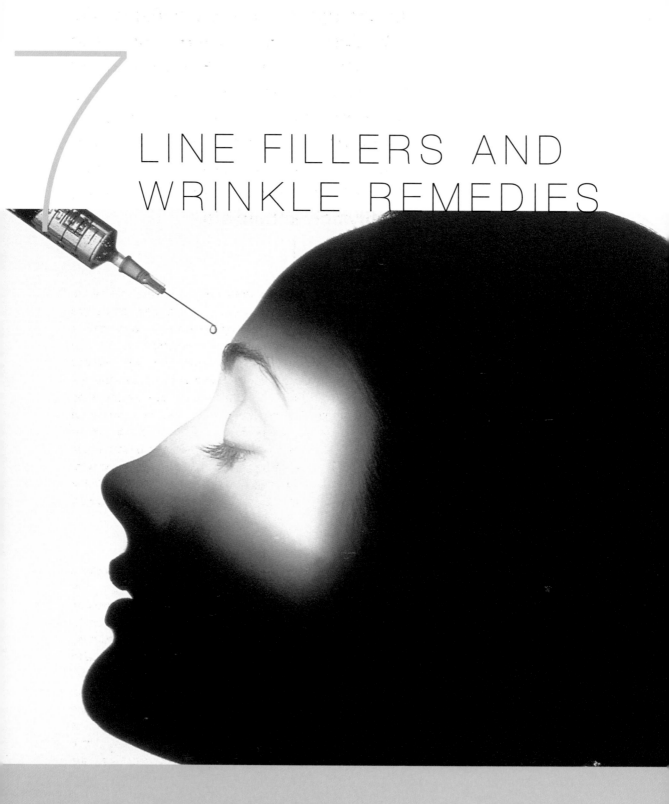

# LINE FILLERS AND WRINKLE REMEDIES

**As we age our dermis deflates, the full lips of our youth thin and expression lines become permanent furrows. The quickest, neatest way of remedying these age-related changes is simply to refill and replenish. The procedures are quick, virtually painless and the results gratifyingly immediate.**

# after several

decades of squinting and smiling, frowning and puckering-up, the facial muscles which govern such movements take their toll on your weakening (perhaps sun-challenged dermis) and the creases which once faded rapidly from view become permanently etched into your face. Of course, a lightly corrugated pair of crow's feet can indicate a happy history but some of the 'expression' lines or marks of past events we

**The reason most patients now cite for 'having something done' is to divest themselves of age-related expression marks that they feel make them look mean or miserable.**

end up with are less becoming. The pockmarks left by severe spots can ruin the look of an otherwise healthy complexion or thinning lips can cause a relatively line-free face to look more mature than it need. Similarly, a recalcitrant frown furrow can mar your naturally good-humoured demeanour and a pair of marionette lines (the ones that descend from the corners of your mouth towards your chin) can make even those who don't mind getting older look glum.

If you are generally happy with your skin tone, but just have one or two deep lines, lips that are deflating with age (or were always too thin) or scars you wish you could plump back out, it may be that all you need is a bit of filler. Without wanting to sound glib about any cosmetic procedure, it is the case that line filling injections are one of the quickest and simplest ways of improving an ageing or damaged face. I and many of my colleagues usually find that while patients are relieved to have a life-threatening mole removed or their spots cured, it is having their lines filled or their lips plumped which often brings the biggest smiles to their face.

### Filling agents

The concept of injecting substances to plump out lines and wrinkles has been around for over 30 years. As with many cosmetic procedures, the idea for them came out of the plastic surgeon's reconstructive work and indeed many of the latest fillers still do. Those fillers available divide into temporary and permanent treatments. Many patients are encouraged to dip their first toe into the cosmetic pool because fillers such as collagen and hyaluronic acid gels don't last (indeed, their very impermanence is one of their safety features) For those who don't want the inconvenience or cost of touch-ups, or those who have had too many of them and want to move on, there are now some safe, reversible and highly effective permanent options.

## The temporary fillers
### Collagen

This is without doubt the best known of all the fillers, largely because it has been around for so long and so many people have been very successfully treated with it.

In the early 1970s biochemists and physicians at Stanford University in California were looking for alternatives to skin grafts in plastic reconstructive surgery. They hit upon the idea of purifying animal collagen to replace the natural human variety – which is remarkably similar. Purified bovine collagen was first used on human subjects in 1976. When this type of collagen is injected into skin depressions or furrows it doesn't take over the role of the natural variety, but effectively fills the gaps created by time and tide.

**Used for:** There are two versions made, Zyderm and Zyplast. The former is a lighter mixture better suited to finer lines such as those around the eye area, the latter is denser and more suitable to fill heavier lines such as around lips and in the naso-labial folds (or smile lines). Zyplast is also useful for plumping out depressed acne scars.

**spot check**

If you are having your lips augmented you might like to bring a picture of what your lips used to look like, or indeed someone else's lips, as a visual aid for your physician. This is useful because it means that neither of you need rely on your powers of description and there is less chance of miscommunication.

### The procedure:

Collagen has a 3–4 per cent allergy risk and if you are one of the susceptible few you will not be able to have collagen injections. You will therefore be required to undergo two allergy tests up to two months beforehand. These involve injecting tiny blobs of collagen into the skin of the inside of your forearm. You will also have to answer questions about any medical conditions you may have that may preclude collagen treatment.

Four weeks later, on the day of your appointment, you will come to the clinic up to an hour before the procedure to have some anaesthetizing cream or gel applied. You will have discussed with your physician exactly what you want. If I, or my patient is in any doubt about what and how much is needed I will always treat the area conservatively – it's always possible to come back for more.

The needle is very small, and it is loaded with some local anaesthetic so while you may feel a little pin-prick, you should not feel too much discomfort as the collagen goes in. It is injected into the upper dermal levels – where all your own collagen is. The procedure may take between 10 minutes and half and hour.

**Afterwards:** You may experience some swelling due either to the local anaesthetic or to a degree of overcorrection – some of the water content in the mix is absorbed within days of the injection. If you bruise very easily you may also have some light bruising.

**Possible risks:** Some people are allergic to collagen but you can become allergic to it at any time. One of my patients, a woman in her 50s who has had four injections of collagen over the past six years suddenly developed an allergic reaction.

You can also get a poor result if the collagen is injected too low in the dermis or even into the subcutis – it will then disappear very rapidly. If you have had cold sores in the past the injection may spark an outbreak. Your physician will probably ask you, but it's wise to remember to tell him so that you can use an anti-viral medication to prevent an attack.

Very, very rarely, the injection site can develop a small scab, some skin shedding or even more rarely, a small ulcer, all of which could leave a scar.

**Duration:** With people whose faces show a lot of ageing-related changes and whose dermis is already quite weak, the collagen may last as little as two to three months. This is true, too, of areas of high activity – in the upper lips, for instance, if you are a smoker. In younger skins and areas which don't move much – say in cheek scars – you might expect your collagen filler to last up to 18 months.

## Hyaluronic acid gel

This is a new filler which I have been using in the UK for over two years but which has yet to be approved for use in the US (red tape rather than safety concerns is causing the delay). Hylaform and Restylene are the tradenames of this viscoelastic form of hyaluronic acid. Originally developed to fill the orbital eye area after injury and to replace lost synovial fluid in the joints of arthritis patients, hyaluronic acid is a natural skin humectant (or water holder). It is a component of NMF (our skin's natural moisturizing factor) which helps to keep the skin supple, hydrated and cushioned. It is also a precursor to collagen. The hyaluronic acid that goes into hylan B gels are extracted from cock's combs, (as is the hyaluronic acid that goes into many of the more expensive moisturizers). Just as with collagen, it is important that vegetarians are aware of the animal source of this filler.

**Used for:** Hyaluronic acid is an alternative to Zyplast as it is a thicker substance and well suited to deeper facial lines. Company literature states that the substance is virtually non-allergenic but my own personal experience suggests otherwise. I believe its allergy rate to be just below that of collagen (ie about 2 per cent). The disadvantage is that there is no thinner form of the gel so it can't be used for very fine lines and with no anaesthetic in the mix, separate injections must be given if required.

**Possible risks:** The chances of an allergic reaction are possibly higher than first thought. It is my belief that allergy testing should be performed as for collagen (see above). There can also be some mild swelling at the injection site which lasts for two to three days maximum.

The procedure, after effects, risks and duration are almost exactly the same as for collagen.

## Fat transfer

This procedure involves using fat either specifically removed for the operation or during liposuction, from another part of your body.

**Used for:** If you have very deep smile lines, sunken cheeks or very deep acne scars your best, and really only, option is to have these areas filled with your own body fat. There are both advantages and disadvantages to using your own tissue. The advantage, obviously, is that there is no chance of any allergic reaction or rejection. The disadvantage is that you first have to have the fat extracted from elsewhere.

**The procedure:** Before you can have the fat injected, it must first be 'harvested'. This is done by mini-tumescent liposuction. Under local anaesthetic, a tiny, fine needle is inserted, usually into the abdomen or flanks ('love handles') of men and thighs of women (only one of my patients has had to go home to put on weight before the procedure). A solution of local anaesthetic, epinephrine (a vaso constrictor) and bicarbonate of soda is included in the needle to inhibit stinging. The fat is then withdrawn through the same needle. Sometimes a single suture (stitch) is required which will stay in for about a week.

What fat isn't needed immediately is carefully labelled, stored in sealed bags and frozen for future use (for up to one year later). What is to be used is loaded into a fine canula – a sort of blunt-ended tube. It scores tunnels in the lower dermis or in the subcutaneous fatty layer beneath and as it is withdrawn tubular grafts of fat are left behind.

**After:** You might have some swelling and/or bruising and some local discomfort which will last a few hours.

**Possible risks:** If the procedure is done properly there shouldn't be a noticeable depression where the fat was taken but there may be some swelling and perhaps even a little temporary discoloration. If injected into parts of the face where there is very little subcutaneous fat – such as lips or around the eyes – there is a risk that you will get lumps and bumps – which is why I don't believe the procedure should be performed there.

**Duration:** Fat transfers lasts longer than the previously mentioned fillers, largely because we tend to use it in areas such as cheeks or scars which aren't subject to much movement. Most patients achieve about a 40–60 per cent persistence over two to three years. In scars it can last longer.

## Isolagen

If you don't like the idea of having bovine collagen injected there is another option – your own. Just approved, Isolagen is the trade name of a new service in which 3 mm biopsies of your own skin are taken – usually from an inconspicuous area – and sent to the company's US laboratory. There, scientists culture your own collagen and the fibroblasts which produce it. Several weeks later the results of your donation and their labours are sent back to your physician.

**Used for:** Isolagen can be used to correct fine smile, frown and lip lines, augment the lips and also fill out concave scars.

**The procedure:** This is similar to that for collagen.

**Afterwards:** The bruising reactions are exactly the same as for bovine collagen.

**Possible risks:** These are the same as for bovine collagen but without the risk of allergy.

**Duration:** According to the company's own literature, Isolagen is longer lasting than bovine collagen but it's a relatively new service and time will tell.

## Botox

Botox is not actually a filler at all but is included here because it is injected into the skin, and because it does smooth out lines. The idea for the use of botulinum toxin came in the 70s from an ophthalmologist Dr Alan Scott in San Francisco who was looking for non-surgical methods of correcting squints and ticks in children. It took about 15 years, however, before dermatologists and plastic surgeons began to see Botox's wrinkle-smoothing capacity.

As its name suggests, Botox is indeed derived from botulinum toxin. A fantastically dilute and highly purified version of the very same bug that causes life-threatening gastric upsets, it is injected into the muscles which cause crow's feet, the folds of a frown or those that cause excessive lip pursing. There is no effect on the central nervous system because the toxin remains locked in the muscle into which it is

Before and after treatment

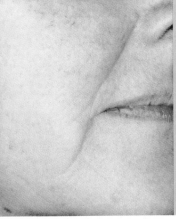
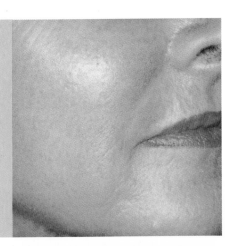

A 44-year-old-female with **lower facial lines** before (A) and after (B) treatment

**treatment:** Fat transfer using patient's own fat harvested from her lower abdomen and injected into the lower face lines

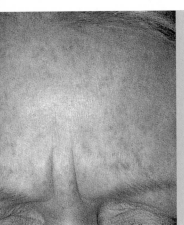
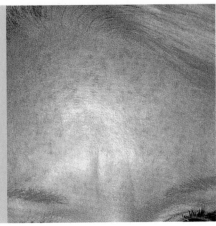

A 59-year-old female with **frown lines** before (A) and after (B) treatment

**treatment:** two Botox injections for lower forehead frown lines

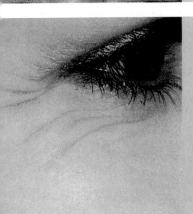
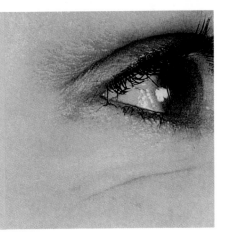

A 32-year-old female with **'crows feet'** before (A) and after (B) treatment

**treatment:** one Botox injection

injected. Gradually, over eight to ten days after your procedure the flow of nerve signals to the muscle is staunched. No longer able to pull on the skin in the way that caused the dermal trench to form, the line is either softened or completely eradicated. The effect is temporary, however, and after three to eight months, the nerves eventually regain their ability to receive and transmit signals. Botox has really revolutionized the treatment and prevention of line formation and is fast becoming the most popular procedure performed.

**Used for:** Botox is now being used to paralyse the muscles that cause creased foreheads – both frown and horizontal lines, eye, upper lip, marionette areas and sometimes the neck. Botox is also being increasingly used by doctors to help alleviate the muscular spasm often associated with Bell's and cerebral palsy and is now being investigated for the relief of tension headaches and migraine.

**The procedure:** For at least the first time you have Botox your physician will probably attach an EMG (electromyogram) to the area to ensure the precise placement of the needle into the muscle. Then the solution is injected into the muscle, probably in several places to ensure that all areas of the muscles are hit. There is no anaesthetic in the solution but apart from some stinging as the solution goes in, the sensation is quite bearable.

It takes up to ten days for the nerves to be completely incapacitated, during which time you may feel nothing at all or perhaps a little light flickering or twitching of the muscle. Many patients are worried that they will look expressionless, but it is our experience that because the face has such an enormously wide range of movements freezing one from your repertoire goes unnoticed. If total lack of

### spot check

An efficient way of prolonging the life of your temporary filler is to have the muscles that caused it in the first place paralysed. An injection of Botox at least two weeks before that of your chosen filler will relax the muscles around the line for several months and can double or even treble the life of your filler.

movement is still a concern, the dosage and depth of the injection can be adjusted simply to weaken the muscle rather than paralyze it completely.

**Afterwards:** If you bruise easily you may have some light marks which will take two or three days to fade. Equally there may be some slight swelling at the injections sites. Occasionally patients complain of a headache.

**Possible risks:** There is as yet no evidence of allergy – certainly after injecting myself, my wife, my co-author, some of my staff and several thousand patients I have yet to see one case of allergy. The only complication can be a slight droop of one eyelid, but in my experience a less than 0.5 per cent risk. It resolves itself within two weeks. There is, however, the reverse risk that you may be resistant to the toxin. Some people may have unknowingly had a sub-clinical bout of botulism which has left them with antibodies to it.

**Duration:** In the first instance, the paralysis lasts only about three to four months, slightly longer with horizontal forehead lines. We are now finding, however, that with each subsequent dose the time lengthens. I (Dr Lowe) have had eight injections over the last 4 years and now only need one every year.

## Semi-permanent fillers
### Alloderm

One of the newer types of filler, Alloderm is a decellurized collagenous graft (or in basic terms a bit of treated skin taken from a cadaver). Sourced from a skin bank, the skin is processed by removing the non-collagen content, purifying the collagen, then drying it into sheets which your physician can cut and shape according to needs – small and round for scars or long and slim for lines or lips.

**Used for:** It is made primarily for reconstructive plastic surgery but has proved to be very useful to the dermatologic surgeon wanting to raise saucer-shaped acne scars and reshape lips (although I prefer Softform for the latter, see below).

**The procedure:** Alloderm arrives in your dermatologist's clinics in desiccated sheets. Half an hour before it is required the sheets are floated in saline until they expand, then they are cut to the size and shape of the scar or rolled into the required shape. Alloderm's insertion into the skin requires minor 'surgery', where a scalpel is used to allow access to the dermal/subcutal junction where it is laid.

**Afterwards:** Anaesthetizing injections need to be given to the patient, so there can be some swelling afterwards.

**Possible risks:** The tissue used has been treated to minimize the risk of rejection but it is still theoretically possible that your body could recognize it as foreign matter. The implant can also move within the skin. I always tether the implant, in place with one

stitch. There is also still a risk of infection at the point of insertion.

**Duration:** It was hoped that because the skin uses the Alloderm implant to grow into that the results would be permanent, but this is not proving to be the case. However, particularly in the case of scars, the results will last from 18 months to three or four years.

## Permanent fillers
### Softform

If you have had collagen and been disappointed at how long it lasted; if you've also tried hyaluronic acid gels and watched them be reabsorbed, or if you are generally fed up with the time and money you have to spend on regular touch ups, you may want to move onto something more permanent. Or you may simply want to try this type of filler first. Softform is a new treatment for the correction of deeper lines and for lip enhancement. Rather than being injected, it is surgically implanted but requires only two small incisions a couple of millimetres long at either end of the line, or lips, being treated.

Softform is essentially Gortex that has been rendered less porous so that skin tissue doesn't infiltrate it. This means that the implant can be easily removed at a later date, if required.

Because the implant itself is a hollow tube, however, new tissue of your own does grow into the centre of it which helps it anchor in place. It is also now becoming apparent that this new tissue remains even if, for whatever reason, the implant is removed, leaving you with more than you started out with.

**Used for:** Naso labial (smile) lines, marionette lines, frown lines and upper and lower lip augmentation. It is useful as a preventative aid for those who are developing upper lip lines as the increased implant actually prevents the excessive pursing action which causes them.

**spot check**

Those having permanent implants admit they take some getting used to. But after a few months most say they've forgotten they are there. They also worry about how their partners might respond to them, how they will fare during what's colloquially known as the 'kissability test'. I know of none who has yet failed it.

**The procedure:** You may be sedated, will certainly be given a local anaesthetic and may benefit from a ring block – total knocking out of the nerves in the area. Your physician will mark the entry and exit incisions. The trocar, a sort of scalpel-ended surgical plunger containing the tubular implant, is inserted from one end to the other and as the trocar is withdrawn the implant is left in its place. The ends are tapered and tucked back in and the incisions closed and stitched.

**Afterwards:** The anaesthesia should ensure that you do not feel too much discomfort, but it will be responsible for some swelling. However, the results of the implant are immediately visible – something that many patients find very gratifying.

**Risks:** As with all surgical incisions there is the risk of infection. This can be minimized by keeping the area clean and by using antibiotic/antiseptic medications. In most patients the incisions produce imperceptible scars and if doing lips these can be hidden within the vermilion border. Some patients however, may develop larger scars. Those with a tendency to hypertrophic or keloid scarring should not be treated. Sometimes the implant can shift position if the new tissue doesn't grow into it quickly enough. This is more likely if you are older or your skin is severely photodamaged because its repair and growth mechanisms are slower.

There are further permanent fillers available, none of which I use for reasons given below. They are not, therefore, discussed in any detail.

**Artecol** is a mixture of collagen and an acrylic cement used in dental and reconstructive surgery. It can feel quite hard in the skin. Even with surgery its removal is almost impossible.

**Gortex** is a very tough but porous material. Skin tissue grows its way into the Gortex matrix making it very difficult to remove, and there is quite a high incidence of infection or rejection making removal necessary. It is exactly this that caused it to be banned in the US in late 1998.

**Gold** There has recently been a fashion, particularly in Europe, for the use of gold filament. However, there is a lack of scientific data to support its use. It can feel unnaturally hard under the skin and there is a possibility of allergic reaction that would necessitate its removal. Extracting very fine threads used, however, is not easy.

## Silicone

Silicone has been used by some physicians for over 30 years to correct naso-labial lines and scars. It is not, however, approved for such use in the US and I do not use it in the UK. There is no evidence, in my opinion, to support the claim that silicone can affect the immune system, but there is enough litigation alone to lead to its disapproval in the US.

Injected droplet by droplet, it was originally thought that enough granulated collagen and fibrous tissue formed around the foreign silicone beads, encapsulating it and locking it in place. However, time has shown that silicone can migrate – especially from around fine-skinned areas – or cause allergic reactions. In the past many allergies were attributable to the use of poor-grade silicone; nevertheless, it is still possible for delayed reactions to occur, sometimes many years after injection. Any delayed reaction – which induces redness and disfiguring lumpiness – usually necessitates silicone's removal, but the substance is notoriously difficult to extract without damaging surrounding tissue. Long-term cortisone therapy is often needed to control the inflammation. Conversely, it's also possible for the body to reject the substance, pushing the tiny beads out through the skin's surface.

## Case study 1

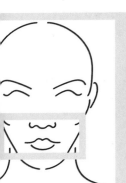

| | |
|---|---|
| Patient: | **Diana** |
| Age: | **47** |
| Problem: | **Thinning lips and depressed scar** |
| Procedure: | **Hylaform** |
| Cost of treatment: | **£350/$580** |
| Result: | **Augmentation of lips lasting 4–6 months and elevation of scar, lasting 18 months** |

### The dermatologist's story

Diana originally came seeking treatments for a depressed scar, but mentioned she was unhappy with the shape of her lips. We decided to treat the lips as well as her scar as I felt that balancing out her top and bottom lips would help draw the eye away from the scar. I chose to treat Diana with a hyaluronic acid gel filler as it was the first time she had had any such treatment. It's easy, safe, and quick to use, and because it's temporary it gives her the opportunity to see if she likes the results secure in the knowledge that if she doesn't they will disappear.

She came to the office to have an anaesthetizing cream applied an hour before, then we injected local anaesthetic into the area to be treated. When the area was numb I injected the Hylaform into the upper dermis, along the length of the lip and the scar. As the needle withdrew a length of gel was left in its wake. The amount used depends on the level of correction the patient desires. Diane wanted very little so I injected very conservatively.

### The patient's story

I didn't like the way a scar left by a cold sore pulled down one corner of my mouth. People kept asking me whether I was unhappy. I went to inquire about having it corrected, and thought I might as well have my thinning lips dealt with at the same time as the same filler could be used.

I went in early to have anaesthetizing cream applied and then had local anaesthetizing injections. I wouldn't say the injections were pain-free; the anaesthetic and the gel injections made my eyes water but it was bearable. I went home with a slightly swollen and bruised face, and I did think 'what have I done?', but two days later it had all calmed down.

I told a couple of friends what I had done, but no one else noticed the difference – not even my husband. But I did. I felt better. I no longer look down in the mouth and my top lip is just that little bit fuller and younger-looking. I will have Hylaform injections again, and perhaps after that consider a more permanent option.

## Case study 2

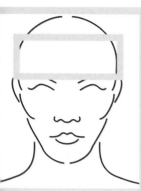

| | |
|---|---|
| Patient: | **Polly** |
| Age: | **34** |
| Problem: | **Frown lines** |
| Procedure: | **Botox** |
| Cost of treatment: | **£175/$290** |
| Result: | **Paralysis of corrugator muscle lasting 3 months (for first injection, longer for subsequent treatments)** |

### The dermatologist's story

Polly had inherited a tendency to glabellar furrows (frown marks), hastened by growing up under the harsh Antipodean sun and spending a lot of time doing outdoor sports. She was a good candidate for Botox because she was a healthy patient and not on any medications or any of the muscle-relaxant drugs which can inhibit Botox, her eyebrows were symmetrical and she had a well-developed corrugator muscle.

In fact, Botox is really the only option to treat frown lines. Fillers such as Zyplast, the thicker collagen mix, should not be injected into the forehead as it can seep into the small blood vessels which run through this area and cause ulceration. Permanent fillers and implants risk being visible as lumps because of the closeness of the bone to the skin.

After informing her of the 1/400 chance of slight eyelid droop which usually only lasts two weeks, I attached an EMG (electromyogram) to ensure I was targeting the strongest area of the muscle and injected the Botox at five sites. I advised her that with such a strong corrugator muscle as hers the effects would probably last only three months and that in order to retain the smoothing results it is a good idea to have regular top-ups before the furrows return.

### The patient's story

I've always hated the great trench that cleaves my forehead in two and have always worn a fringe to cover it up. When I walk along the street and the wind blows my fringe aside all I can see reflected in windows is an angry scowl. Botox seemed the perfect entry into the cosmetic arena for me, largely because the effects are temporary.

The injections hurt a great deal less than some inoculations I've had. I couldn't wait for the toxin to take effect. Over the next eight to 10 days I could feel the faintest flickering as the paralysis set in and eventually, try as I might I couldn't frown. Over the next few weeks the line softened immeasurably. I could see it still but it was completely flat instead of deeply entrenched. I no longer cared if a breeze blew away my fringe. I loved not having to worry about whether I was squinting in the sunshine and causing a deeper frown line.

I had worried slightly that I might look slightly expressionless, but no one noticed I wasn't scowling at them any more. (I found it's perfectly possible to show displeasure without frowning.) Now the very temporary nature of Botox, which attracted me to it in the first place, is the thing I most regret.

## Case study 3

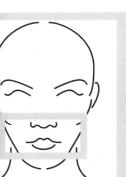

| | |
|---|---|
| Patient: | **Claire** |
| Age: | **57** |
| Problem: | **Thinning lips and upper lip lines** |
| Procedure: | **Softform implant** |
| Cost of treatment: | **£1000/$1650** |
| Result: | **Permanent lip augmentation** |

### The dermatologist's story

The plump fatty cushion that gives young lips their volume had reduced with age leaving this patient with thinned lips. I recommended the safe Softform permanent filler as this patient did not want the expense of repeated temporary fillers. This filler also gives the lips more resilience and prevents the upper lip lines from deepening. The procedure is a surgical one but is performed under local anaesthesia. After marking the position of the implant and the insertion incisions and dulling the area with some anaesthetizing cream I injected some local anaesthetic. I prepared two upper and one lower implant, and then performed a ring block – a complete block of the nerve tissue in the entire nose and mouth area.

The incisions are made with a 4 mm (⅛ in) cutting needle and the implant-bearing trocar was inserted at the lower dermal level along the lip. I then stretched the skin and the implant to ensure that the tissue was evenly draped over it. The ends of the implant were then tapered off, tucked back in and closed with one or two stitches. The procedure took about half an hour.

Claire was able to apply make-up immediately and go back to work. She came back in five days later to have the stitches removed.

### The patient's story

I never had very full lips but they were deflating with each year. The corners of my mouth had turned down and I was developing lines over my upper lips. With a deep frown line, too, I felt that even when relaxed I looked angry or miserable.

I was the first person in the UK to have Softform but I talked to Dr Lowe and, hearing that it has been used in arterial surgery for over 25 years, I was reassured. We discussed a temporary filler but I didn't want to spend the money or time on regular top ups. Fat transfer wasn't an option for me either as Dr Lowe told me I didn't have enough!

I came in during my lunch break and had local anaesthetizing injections. All I felt was some slight tugging and pulling. Immediately afterwards I went back to work – I wasn't in any pain but just felt a little battered. The swelling was worst on the third day, but I had no bruising and the swelling decreased over the next two days. The stitches healed quickly with no problems.

Those who haven't seen me in a while tell me I look really well and happy. My lips are slightly fuller, my Cupid's bow is more defined, and the corners of my mouth turn very slightly up instead of down. And now, having had Botox, too, for my frown lines, my expression is altogether more pleasant.

# 8 PEELING BACK THE YEARS

**Maybe you feel your skin has lost its youthful patina. Maybe you don't want to go under the knife but would like a fresher, younger-looking complexion. A resurfacing procedure will remove your crinkled skin and incite a smoother one to grow in its place.**

# the peeling principle

While the processes and the equipment vary, the aim of all peeling or resurfacing procedures is the same – to remove skin layers. Unlike some of our other organs, our skin possesses remarkable

## Taking off the skin's outer layer in essence wipes out a generation of epidermal cells with UV-damaged memories.

recuperative powers. The principle is similar to pruning: pare back the skin layers to get better growth. If you remove the epidermis, it literally grows back. Indeed, so keen is your skin to regenerate, that it does so without bothering to replicate some of the added extras it developed during its lifetime – the wrinkles and furrows, blotches and dark spots. Taking off the skin's outer layer in essence wipes out a generation of epidermal cells with UV-damaged memories.

The net result, once the healing process is complete, is not only a younger-looking complexion, but one that is, to all intents, younger; the epidermal cells are new, and the dermis contains more of the substances that make it firm, plump and elastic.

### The types

Resurfacing procedures divide into three different types: light, medium and deep.

- If you're after a marginally smoother-feeling and slightly brighter-looking complexion, or you simply want a low-key introduction to such procedures, your physician may suggest. a light peel.

- If you have signs of photo-damage – a rough, dull complexion, light wrinkles, dark sun or 'age' spots – a medium peel can freshen your skin tone, smooth out wrinkles and erase solar lentigo (age spots).

- If your skin is severely sun-damaged with lots of deep wrinkles, a bumpy shiny appearance (elastosis), and mottling, a deep procedure can all but wipe them from your face.

### spot check

Many commercial skin clinics are now boasting peeling procedures – laser resurfacing in particular – as the safe, easy alternative to a facelift. If you have lots of sagging skin, however, nothing short of the surgeon's scalpel will divest you of it.

123

## The methods

There are three different techniques used by physicians to improve the look and tone of the sun damaged and aged complexion:

- Chemical peeling

- Dermabrasion

- Laser resurfacing

Chemical peeling involves the painting on of a caustic solution such as glycolic acid, trichloracetic acid, or the very extreme phenol to remove skin layers. Dermabrasion involves abrading away the upper layers of skin with a scouring device. The newest variation on the resurfacing theme involves high-tech pulsed beam lasers. Their computer controlled precision is unparalleled and the shrinking of collagen fibres which seems to occur during healing generates a firming, lifting effect that can, in some patients, obviate the need for surgery.

## The resurfacing physician or surgeon

It is important to be aware that even in the very best hands, people's bodies are infinitely variable. No physician can be 100 per cent certain of exactly how each skin will react to a procedure. It is generally accepted that a 30 per cent or below glycolic acid solution is unlikely to carry any risk of permanent damage. As a result, many beauty salons are now offering such treatments. However, these barely rate as a chemical 'peel' as they do not so much peel away layers of skin as remove more skin cells than would normally be removed by a really vigorous face scrub.

Medium and deep resurfacing procedures – whether they are chemically, physically or laser induced – should not be undertaken lightly. Their aim, after all, is the annihilation of the outer layer

**spot check**

Most dermatologists will recommend that you should give up smoking for a period before and after undergoing a resurfacing procedure. Because smoking constricts the capillaries, reduces the flow of oxygen to the skin tissue and also depletes vitamin C reserves, it may jeopardize the formation of new collagen and so prolong the healing process.

of your face. You, and your physician must be convinced that you have a sufficiently good case for treatment. Equally important is that the procedure is carefully matched to the level of damage present and the desired result. Disreputable clinics are often keen to treat anyone who can pay.

When investigating any resurfacing treatment, make sure that you know all the facts – good and bad. The two pages of 'risks and possible side effects' you are handed may not make for encouraging reading but the absence of such material is more worrying.

You, and your physician must be convinced that you have a sufficiently good case for treatment. Equally important is that the procedure is carefully matched to the level of damage present and the desired result.

## Before and after treatment

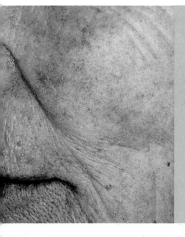
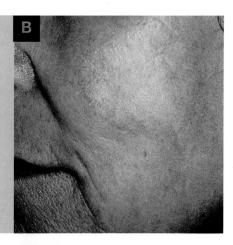

A 62-year-old woman with **severely sun-damaged skin** before (A) and after (B) treatment

**treatment:** skin rejuvenating with an ultrapulsed carbon-dioxide laser

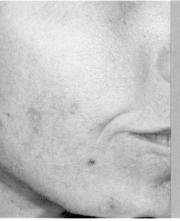
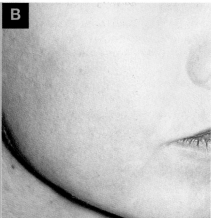

A 42-year-old woman with **post-acne scarring and lines** before (A) and after (B) treatment

**treatment:** tretinoin cream for 6 weeks and one TCA peel (25 per cent)

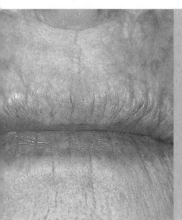
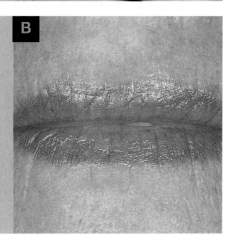

A 58-year-old female with **rhytides** before (A) and after (B) treatment

**treatment:** skin rejuvenating with an ultrapulsed carbon-dioxide laser

# Chapter Eight

## You and your resurfacing procedure

**Whether you opt for a light chemical peel over your whole face or a deep laser resurfacing over your top lip only, the before, during and aftercare process is similar. The deeper the peel, the longer and more difficult the recovery period may be, but the benefit is that the effects are more marked.**

## Finding a qualified physician

- Ask about his or her medical qualifications and memberships of which boards. Look for specialized training in dermatology, cosmetic surgery, laser surgery and/or plastic surgery. Disreputable clinics may employ general practitioners with no dermatological or specialist cosmetic surgery training. If you don't know what constitutes specialist training, check with your doctor who can find out for you.

- Find out how long the physician has been performing your chosen procedure.

- Ask how many patients he or she has treated.

- Ask to see before and after photos of patients treated

- Ask to speak personally to one or more patients.

- Ensure that your treatment will be carried out by, or under the supervision of, the physician with whom you have your consultation. Some clinics hand over the actual treatment to staff with no medical or specialist training.

## Be wary of

- Magazine advertisements, especially those that feature seductive imagery. In Britain there are some very good private clinics but these tend to be attached to well-known hospitals and have NHS consultant-status surgeons or dermatologists operating from them.

- Promises of instant rejuvenation, facelifts without surgery, or any procedure which claims to offer maximum results for minimal cost – financial or personal.

**Note:** Remember that commercial clinics can advertize their services while individual consultant dermatologists are forbidden by the General Medical Council from doing so. Also bear in mind, too, that provided they do not claim to have medical qualifications, anyone can set up a clinic.

### Before

The preparation of your skin is vitally important before treatment and can be the key to the final result. For four weeks prior to a superficial treatment you will be encouraged to use topical glycolic, Retin-A, perhaps ascorbic acid preparation, and if you have very dark skin, lightening agents to help prevent dark patches forming as your skin heals. The action of these agents will:

- Ensure the removal any build up of dead, horny cells from the stratum corneum which might impede the progress of the peeling chemical.

- Help ensure a uniform result.

- Speed up cell turnover in readiness for the repair process.

- Lighten any pigmented patches and decrease the likelihood of any forming after the peel.

**You should also:**

- Stay out of the sun. The irregular formation of melanin could leave you with uneven brown patches.
- Stop smoking. Smoking contributes to free radical damage and starves the skin of oxygen and so prolongs the healing process.

**Note:** In some cases, the use of Retin-A and alpha hydroxy acid preparations alone improve the complexion to the point where both the patient and the physician decide that a peel is no longer necessary.

If you are undergoing a medium or deep procedure, this preparative skin care regime will start six weeks before.

It is important that you adhere strictly to the regime, or if you are experiencing problems with it, that you inform your physician. The more rigorous the procedure, the more important the ante-peel care becomes. You and your physician will want to be confident that your stratum corneum has been denuded of its horny build up to allow the chemical to penetrate uniformly, and that your cell turnover is right up to speed so that you achieve optimum, even healing. Indeed, if the pre-resurfacing treatment doesn't achieve the sort of smooth, even skin texture your physician is looking for, it's quite possible that he or she may not wish to perform the procedure.

Before a deep resurfacing it is wise to make some arrangements for your aftercare. While after a light glycolic acid peel you might go home or back to work, you will need to be driven home after a deep peel. You will feel groggy, and probably have a fair amount of discomfort, and may have dressings on your face for several days. You should not, nor will you want to, move around much for five to seven days so, if possible, arrange to have someone to help you out.

On the day of the procedure, wear a top that you can unbutton to take off when you get home. Patients who have forgotten this piece of advice report only momentary regret for a favourite cashmere sweater as they reach for the scissors rather than risk pulling it over their tender face. If you are nervous about the procedure, you may be given a sedative to help you sleep the night before.

## During

Your face is cleansed – dry or sensitive skin with soap, normal skin with alcohol and oily skin with acetone – to strip the skin of sebum which might impede the acid penetration or interfere with the laser beam. This is particularly important in greasy skins. However, the level of degreasing must be taken into account by the physician, particularly with chemical peels. Heavy or aggressive degreasing can significantly increase the action of the solution to the extent that a relatively light 50 per cent concentration solution can produce a medium-depth peel effect. This is generally considered an advantage as a better result can then be achieved by using a less concentrated solution. However, if it is attempted by inexperienced hands, the unexpected transformation of a light peel into a medium one might not make for a happy ending.

**If you are having a chemical peel,** the solution will be swabbed or painted on and you will experience a stinging, burning or prickling sensation. The acid is left on the skin for between one and seven minutes during which time the use of a cool air fan can alleviate some of the discomfort. The physician will be carefully monitoring your skin, looking for the level of redness that indicates the depth of acid penetration. At the end of the maximum time, your face is sponged with ice water to neutralize the acid.

**If you opt for dermabrasion** this can be performed under local anaesthetic, or a local with some oral sedation, but is more likely to be conducted under full general anaesthetic as the treatment is painful.

If you are having your entire face dermabraded the process might take up to two hours, if your cheeks only are to be done it make take one hour, and if it's only your upper lip to be treated it may all be over in 30 minutes.

**If you are going under the laser** you will be given a mixture of oral sedatives and local anaesthetic or perhaps be put under conscious sedation by an anaesthetist and have local anaesthetizing injections in each area 10 minutes before it is treated. (Most dermatologists and surgeons prefer to avoid a general anaesthetic whenever possible because it can be more risky.)

The area to be treated is then mapped out and your eyes covered with laser shields to protect them from the intense light. Your physician will wear both eye goggles and a mask over his mouth and nose to protect him or herself from inhaling the skin vapour (it is theoretically possible for diseases such as the HIV virus to be transmitted via inhalation).

The laser beam itself is emitted from a small 'pen' to produce a tiny pinpoint of light, or from a computerized handpiece that is programmed to stipple minute spots of the beam in a variety of different patterns that range from a 1 cm (⅓ in) square of 100 dots to triangles or hexagons of dots. If using the computerized handpiece, the physician will choose the pattern according to the size and shape of the area to be treated and may vary the pattern for different parts of the face.

When the laser is fired there is a flash of light and the skin surface yields a puff of vaporized tissue.

The level of discomfort or pain varies with the level of sedation and/or local anaesthetic given.

The whole area to be treated will be 'painted' with, initially, just one pass of the laser. If there are any deeper lines and wrinkles, the physician may pass the laser over again. The edges surrounding the part being treated may have to be feathered using less energy to avoid a discernible line.

Although several layers of skin are being removed, even the deeper laser treatments are virtually bloodless as the light beam cauterizes the affected blood vessels.

## Immediately afterwards

After a superficial glycolic acid peel your face may be rosy pink to red, or you may notice little difference. In some cases there may be a faint whitish discoloration over certain areas where the acid has caused a separation of some of the superficial cell layers – a sort of blister. Mild swelling may also be noted. These are all normal reactions.

After a deeper chemical peel or laser resurfacing you may be white or yellowish where the skin cells and collagen have been seared. Your pale face will rapidly turn pink or red as an increased blood supply rushes to the rescue. It will also be swollen. Pink and puffy is how you will remain for about 48 hours to a couple of weeks depending on the treatment. One to two days after your peel you might be hard-pressed to find a line anywhere as all your wrinkles are puffed out beyond recognition.

After dermabrasion your face will feel raw and be hidden under dressings which will need changing frequently. You will be sent home with instructions for the care of your healing skin including all or some of the following:

- Protective moisturizing creams.
- Moist gel dressings.
- Antibiotic medication.
- Anti-viral medication – to deter cold sores.
- Emollient creams to keep the old shedding skin supple and the new skin moist and protected. Apply these regularly.

## Over the next few days

If your peel was very light, you may notice little change. If you underwent a deeper procedure, you will experience more marked skin 'peeling' including a gradual darkening of the 'white' areas which then dry out and peel away. After the deepest peel your face will become scaly but do not pick at the scabbing as this increases the risk of infection, causes uneven healing and spoils the changing skin. Medication can be prescribed to alleviate it. Keep your skin moist and supple by washing, applying moist dressings or bland oils or moisturizers. As healing progresses, your face may itch. Do not expose your face to the sun without a sunscreen for at least six weeks. To do so increases the risk of irregularly pigmented patches. However, you won't be able to apply sunscreen until the epidermis has regenerated (about 2–3 weeks after treatment). In the mean-time, cover up and/or stay indoors .When your epidermis has healed sufficiently so that you can apply make-up and regular creams, begin using an SPF15-20 day cream. Wearing a daily sun-screen will help maintain the results of your peel and may take away the need for subsequent ones.

## Potential complications resurfacing procedures

- Burning, itching and/or swelling can be persistent in some patients. It can be reduced by using cold compresses (cotton wool pads dipped in icy water). If concerned, check with your physician.
- Temporary hyperpigmentation (excessively dark patches) may occur in some patients with skin types 3 or above despite their best efforts to avoid sunlight. If dark patches do form, bleaching creams can help significantly.
- Some acne lesions may initially be more noticeable and redder. These usually improve within 3 days after the procedure.
- Fine blood vessels of the face are not relieved by peeling and may appear more vibrant. Cosmetics can be used to camouflage these or they can be permanently treated with light electrocautery, with a laser, or by sclerotherapy.
- Rarely, bacterial infections may occur, and if a patient has a predisposition toward herpes simplex (cold sores), these lesions may be precipitated by the procedure. Both conditions, if they develop, can be treated with antibiotic or antiviral medications. It is important, however, to tell your physician as soon as symptoms are noticed so that treatment can begin without delay.
- Scarring is always a possibility, particularly after a deep peel. You can minimise the risk by ensuring you do not allow your skin to dry out or crack.
- Erythema, or redness can persist for up to three months, particularly in fair-skinned patients.

## Chemical skin peels

**Chemical peels use acid solutions to remove, or actively kill off (induce necrosis or denaturing of) a predetermined numbers of the upper layers of skin. Chemical peels have been performed for over 40 years – ever since a Florida beauty therapist revealed to Dr Tom Baker the secret 'fountain of youth' phenol mixture she used on her clients to improve photo-aged skin, smooth scarred complexions, reduce wrinkles, remove pre-cancerous lesions or generally to 'freshen up' a tired complexion.**

The depth and effects of a peel on a person's face is controlled by:

● The chemical used.

● The concentration of the solution.

● The time the solution remains in contact with the skin.

● The preparation of the skin prior to treatment. The depth of peel required depends on the damage the skin shows and the improvement sought by the patient. Sometimes, a combination of peels may be required to achieve the best result. Some patients, for instance, may desire, a deep peel around a very wrinkled mouth but, only a medium or superficial acid peel over their upper face.

### Superficial peels

The two main chemicals involved in such peels are glycolic acid and lower concentrations (up to 15 per cent) of trichloracetic acid, or TCA.

**Glycolic acid** This is the best for superficial peeling of mildly sun damaged skin or complexions showing the first signs of ageing – very fine lines, general dullness of tone, slightly uneven pigment.

**spot check**

Many salons and clinics now offer the so-called lunch-time peels. These very superficial peels offer modest improvements and allow you to go about your normal daily activities because there is no discernible after-effect. The only real inconvenience is to your wallet rather than to your schedule as the results are minimal and short-lived.

The treatment is usually performed with a 30–70 per cent concentration. As you have read, glycolic acid is naturally derived from sugar cane. It is non-toxic and is not absorbed into the body, so cannot cause any systemic side-effects in the same way as chemicals such as phenol. (Note: toxicity can occur if industrial, rather than pure medical grade glycolic acid is used. The use of cheaper industrial grade glycolic acid in disreputable clinics has been reported.)

**Suitable candidates** For many patients, whatever their skin damage, a light peel provides an easy entry into the world of aesthetic dermatology. Unlike a facial, it offers a real – albeit limited – complexion clearing result. But unlike the deeper acting variety, none of the complications or any of the giveaways: no recovery period, no redness, no marked scaling or skin peeling.

Acne sufferers, too, may benefit from a light peel to: help clear present comedones; prevent the build-up of future ones; even out the irregular pigmentation that often accompanies acne; and help increase the penetration of topical treatment such as Retin-A and antibiotic creams.

**What to expect** A smoother, fresher-looking complexion. It's the equivalent of a vigorous face scrub, although preferable because it is now thought that even a very light glycolic acid treatment is registered by the dermis which then produces new collagen.

## Types of peels

| Skin type | for | chemical | recovery | risks | result |
|-----------|-----|----------|----------|-------|--------|
| **LIGHT** | Mild sun damage, general poor skin texture | 30%-70% glycolic acid, or up to 15% TCA | Normal activity (including applying make-up) can usually be resumed immediately | Mild swelling, brown spots, infection (rare), no effect | Minimal to moderate smoothing and/or brightening of complexion |
| **MEDIUM** | Moderate sun damage including noticeable lines and pigmented patches | 20%-35% TCA, Jessner's or combination of 50%-70% glycolic + TCA. Or 50-70% glycolic + Jessner's | 7 days (possible to use concealing make-up after five days) | Temporary hypo-pigmentation, persistent erythema (redness) | Noticeable reduction in depth of wrinkles, removal of brown spots, smoother, clearer complexion |
| **DEEP** | Severe sun damage including deep wrinkles, lax tone, marked brown | 35%-50% TCA or phenol | 3 weeks | Permanent hypo-pigmentation (complete loss of pigment), infection, persistent erythema | Dramatic smoothing of wrinkles, obliteration of pigmented lesions, general bleaching of complexion |

Because there is virtually no risk of permanent damage, 30 per cent of glycolic acid treatments are performed in salons. Superficial glycolic acid peels are referred to as 'lunchtime peels' as people can resume normal activities after treatment.

Glycolic acids work by dissolving the intercellular glue that holds skin cells together thus persuading them to take their leave sooner rather than later. The epidermis then churns out new cells to make up the deficit and the dermis responds by making more collagen and elastin. Biopsies of glycolic acid treated skin show epidermal and dermal renewal.

For best results, three and five light peels are usually prescribed because the effects of each peel are cumulative. Ideally, the peels are repeated at two-weekly intervals to allow sufficient healing between treatments, but not enough time for the stratum corneum to build up a thick barrier of horny cells.

## TCA, or trichloracetic acid

This acid used in up to a 15 per cent solution is classified as a superficial peel, but is a marginally 'deeper' light peel than glycolic. Originally used to treat warts, TCA is not a natural chemical but a synthesized one, similar to acetic acid, (i.e. vinegar). Even at 15 per cent TCA results in a deeper peel because it works differently. Rather than acting on the intercellular glue, the acid infiltrates the cells, denaturing or coagulating its protein content thereby killing it.' As a result, TCA is also very effective in treating mild to moderate pre-cancerous skin lesions such as the small scaly lumps, solar keratoses which glycolic acid won't completely clear.

**Suitable candidates** Because it can clear away solar keratoses and solar lentigo as well as smoothing out fine lines, TCA is first choice for the light peeling of skins displaying early forms of these sun-induced changes. It's usually a better option, too, for patients with oily skins and no history of sensitivities, who generally do not have a marked response to glycolic acid, or for patients disappointed by a glycolic acid treatment.

TCA is also useful for treating hands, forearms and necks which because of lack of protection, often display more marked UV-induced changes.

**What to expect** First, the bad news – TCA causes more stinging and burning which lasts longer. You will not be able to go back to work afterwards as you will look uncomfortably sunburnt and your face will be slightly swollen. Thick skin peeling will continue for several days, and while the skin is healing there is a greater risk of infection and/or complication. Now the good news – you can expect a clearer, brighter skin tone, marked smoothing of fine wrinkles and the removal of most of the scaly and dark patches that brought you to us in the first place.

## Medium peels

A combination of different chemicals are often used to perform medium-depth peels.

## Chemicals used for these peels

- A TCA solution of up to 35 per cent.

- Jessner's solution (named after Dr Max Jessner who perfected the acid treatment being used by a US beauty therapist. It is a combination of 15 per cent resorcinol, a resin-based solvent, plus 15 per cent of both lactic and salicylic acids which loosen up the intercellular glue and permit the resorcinol to get through to the lower epidermal layers.

● A combination of 50–70 per cent glycolic TCA or Jessner's solution. Sometimes two chemicals work better than one. For patients who have had a disappointing result from a single mid-depth peel or for those who are suitable candidates for a deep peel but don't want to go that far, the combination of a glue dissolver and a cell denaturer is often very effective.

**Suitable candidates** If you are displaying the signs of 'moderate' photo damage – you have noticeable lines and wrinkles, obvious brown sun spots and perhaps some thickened areas of waxy-looking skin (known as solar elastosis) – your physician will probably suggest a medium-depth peel. Medium peels are also recommended for those left with small, shallow acne scars.

Patients who choose medium-depth peels are often seeking only a moderate improvement in their complexion, and are happy to retain some gentle lines to give the impression of a face ageing gracefully. They also usually have busy lives so like being able to resume a normal day-to-day routine after about five days, albeit with some camouflaging make-up.

**What to expect** From this depth of peel you can expect a marked softening of your deeper lines, possibly the elimination of some finer ones, and a positive evening out of

### spot check

**With the arrival of resurfacing lasers, deep chemical peels are becoming increasingly redundant. In fact, I haven't performed a phenol peel in nearly a decade. They may still be performed by physicians who have been doing them for years or by those who either don't have access to or have experience of the expensive resurfacing lasers.**

skin tone including the eradication of most of your solar lentigo and solar keratoses. Of course, what most patients want to know is just how many years will be whittled away. Unfortunately, it's impossible to be precise. Certainly, the acid will sear away many of the visible changes in your complexion that have been developing for years, and, as well as improving clarity on the surface, new collagen will grow in the dermis giving a renewed firmness and resilience.

Your skin should be sufficiently healed within about five to seven days to allow you to wear camouflaging make-up but will not be completely healed before about two weeks.

## Deep peels

Normally two main chemicals are used to perform deep peels.

### Chemical solutions used

● 35–50 per cent TCA.
● Phenol, or Baker's phenol, first described in the 1950s by Dr Tom Baker, a Miami plastic surgeon.

**Suitable candidates** Deep peels are suggested when the patient has a severe chronic sun damage (actinic degeneration) and is seeking a really radical rejuvenating result. Anyone considering a deep chemical peel must be made aware of the 6-week pre-treatment skin care routine, the pain involved, and the long, difficult and risk-heavy recovery period. Understandably, this immediately eliminates many potential candidates.

The use of the most radical peeling solution, phenol, or Baker's phenol further limits suitable candidates. It is a corrosive chemical which sears its way through the entire epidermis and most of the dermis and can make a badly damaged complexion smooth again. But, (and it's a big but), phenol has an as-yet-unexplained but nevertheless well-documented effect of robbing the melanocytes of their ability to produce pigment. Even after regeneration, melanocytes never regain this pigment power. As a result, the complexion of phenol treated patients is often like fine porcelain. For this reason, phenol peels are best performed on very fair people with less pigment to lose. They should never be performed on those with skin types 3 or darker on whom a pallid complexion would sit strangely above a brown body, or indeed on those who, despite our best efforts to persuade them otherwise, insist on gaining a deep tan.

Phenol can also cause irregularities in heart beat and for this reason a patient must be attached to a cardiac monitor during, and for several hours after, a phenol peel. Patients with a history of heart trouble, therefore, are unsuitable candidates for phenol peels.

**What you can expect** TCA can help remove fine to moderate lines. Pre-cancerous lesions will also be removed, as will solar lentigo and some shallow scars.

With phenol, you will get the most radical skin-smoothing result possible: removal of even deep furrows. But the price paid for radical results is high. Phenol peeling involves much pain, an increased risk of complications including scarring, a long recovery period, and the likelihood of permanent loss of skin pigment.

Even the most hard-hearted dermatologist admits that applying high-strength TCA, and especially phenol, is agonizingly painful. Local anaesthesia is frequently sufficient but general anaesthesia is sometimes the preferred method of pain control. This, of course, is also risky. Also phenol can cause heart irregularities. A specialist anaesthetist (a further expense) should always be present to monitor the patient undergoing a phenol peel.

## Peeling versus surgery

Many clinics offer chemical or laser peels as an alternative to surgery. In fact, the two procedures offer quite different results. Peeling acts on the skin's surface and should improve the complexion. Surgery removes excess lax skin and can lift gravity-pulled skin into a new position. However, some laser resurfacing can, to an extent, firm and tone the skin by causing contraction of the bundles of collagen and elastin fibres in the dermis. For some patients, this may indeed produce enough of a 'lifting' effect to obviate their desire for surgery. But if there is a lot of slack skin, surgery remains the only option for a radical result. Equally, the end result of surgery can be disappointing if the skin texture is poor. Increasingly, therefore, cosmetic surgeons are following up facial surgery with chemical peels or laser resurfacing procedures to improve the overall final result.

- Combining surgery with lasers or peels is increasingly common practice.

- Minimally invasive procedures such as laser resurfacing, Botulinium toxin (for crow's feet and forehead lines) and filler injections to deep lines may postpone surgery.

## Dermabrasion – the plane truth

**Dermabrasion involves quite simply, but rather gruesomely, abrading or scouring away layers of skin. The dermatologist uses a motor driven sanding wheel armed with a fine grade of silica or a rotating steel brush to destroy – by mulching away – all epidermal layers and often most of the dermis.**

### What is it used for?

Given the new advanced lasers in use today, dermabrasion sounds, and indeed, is, a relatively old-fashioned technique. While it may be the case that the next decade will see lasers push dermabrasion into the dermatological history

> Dermabrasion may be used over the upper lip area to erase the lines which act as frustratingly efficient irrigation channels for lipstick.

books, it remains a useful tool in the physician's anti-ageing arsenal, particularly for small facial scars, that occur from acne, for example.

### Suitable candidates

Because dermabrasion removes all the epidermal layers and most of the dermis, it can smooth away some of the deepest lines. It is often used over the upper lip area only to erase lines which radiate out from the thinning mouth. Such wrinkles are often a source of distress to many women who complain they make them look 'mean mouthed' or give them a pinched expression. They also act as frustratingly efficient irrigation channels for lipstick wearers giving the wearer more of a starburst than rosebud-shaped mouth. Despite the depth to which it goes, dermabrasion is less likely than phenol to destroy all skin pigment.

It's not understood why, but some patients with saucer shaped acne scars benefit more from dermabrasion than laser resurfacing. However, dermabrasion cannot be performed on those who have taken Roaccutane (the oral vitamin-A anti-acne drug) during the last year because the drug works by shrinking the sebaceous gland and this can inhibit normal healing. Indeed, anyone with abnormal wound healing, for example, keloid scarring, is not a suitable patient for dermabrasion as the treatment leaves one big, open, raw, wound.

### What to expect

For upper lip lines there should be a 30–40 per cent reduction in the depth of wrinkles and up to a 70 per cent improvement in the brightness and clarity of skin tone. For acne scars you might get about a 30 per cent improvement in their appearance after each treatment. (Dermabrasion can be repeated after a six month break.)

### spot check

**If patients are thrilled with the latest lasers, dermatologists and plastic surgeons, too, are mostly delighted to be able to hang up their whirring steel brushes in favour of a high-tech wand – not only because lasers are more precise and versatile, but because they are also much less grisly.**

## Laser resurfacing – light years ahead

**The newest cosmetic weapon that is wielded by the dermatologist waging war against wrinkles, sun spots and pre-cancerous lesions is the laser.**

### What it involves

Laser resurfacing, sometimes referred to as 'laser peeling', involves short pulse or rapid-scanning carbon-dioxide ($CO_2$) or the Erbium Yag lasers. They emit intense bursts of light energy lasting only a fraction of a second. As the laser passes the skin, it's energy is absorbed by the water in each cell and is instantly vaporized. The depth and intensity of the energy is computer controlled making them very precise devices.

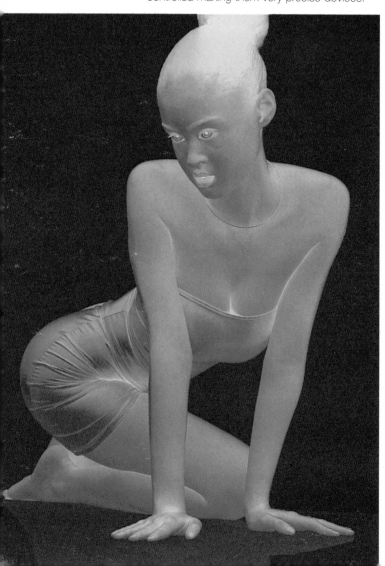

Like so many other medical and cosmetic developments, the wrinkle-smoothing power of the laser was revealed while it was in use for wholly different applications. In the early 1990s, Drs Larry David and Gary Lask of Los Angeles were treating pre-cancerous lesions of the upper lip area with a new pulsed carbon-dioxide device when they noted that as well as clearing the solar keratoses, wrinkles too, were eradicated.

Both the carbon-dioxide ($CO_2$) laser and the Erbium YAG are currently used for skin resurfacing. The Erbium YAG is currently being offered by specialist laser clinics as the safer, gentler of the two devices. Some of their advertizing seems to promise that a short laser treatment will make you look ten years younger. Laser resurfacing, however, is rarely that simple. If it were, you would be unlikely to come away looking weeks younger, let alone years.

The reason some clinics claim the Erbium YAG is 'safer' is because its energy is very efficiently absorbed by the water in your cells, more so than the $CO_2$'s energy. This means there is less chance of deeper heat injury because each pass of the laser removes a thinner layer of cells. However, this efficiency means that the laser continues to vaporize cells with each pass, (unlike the $CO_2$ laser beam, the progress of which is impeded by the skin debris). So the beam is safe, up to a point. If the operator passed over the same bit of skin too many times, however, he or she could easily effect a deeper peel than intended, possibly robbing your skin of pigment and/or scarring it. Nevertheless, the Erbium is popular with some practitioners because of its versatility.

The gentler claim arises from the length of healing time – just one pass of the laser and healing time is down to less than five days. But the fewer the passes, the less radical the result.

The most important thing is that the physician who is performing your procedure is experienced in the use of a wide variety of lasers and techniques so that he or she can choose the right one, or right combination, for you. I use both lasers. Sometimes I use the Erbium YAG for superficial procedures, or the $CO_2$ followed by the Erbium for deep lines or scars which the $CO_2$ can no longer reach.

> It is becoming apparent that improvements often continue in the laser resurfaced face for up to one year after the procedure itself.

### Suitable candidates

If your face is sun damaged with a leathery texture, lines and wrinkles, laxity, thickened areas of skin (solar elastosis), solar lentigo (or 'age' spots) – you might well be a suitable candidate for laser resurfacing.

### What to expect

Laser resurfacing gives a renewed and more youthful complexion. Wrinkles are smoothed, age spots are removed, and the growth of new collagen is stimulated making the skin firmer and younger looking.

Compared to dermabrasion or chemical peeling laser resurfacing carries relatively few risks largely due to the precise nature of the laser and the lack of bleeding. Recovery time too is reduced with most patients. One of my patients who had previously had a chemical peel over her neck and chest was amazed at the speed of healing time when she had her top lip resurfaced with the laser.

A full face resurfacing treatment takes up to two hours, requires a longer healing time, but provides the most dramatic results. In a study performed on 100 women at Dr Lowe's Santa Monica clinic, those who underwent full face resurfacing were generally more satisfied with the results than those who had a limited area treated. This was largely because the erythema (redness) was experienced uniformly all over the face and, therefore, wasn't as noticeable as when it occurred in isolated patches.

It has also been found that a deep laser peel can remove up to 20 years of wrinkles and mottling, a medium one about ten years. What's more, it is becoming apparent that improvements often continue in the laser resurfaced face for up to one year after the procedure itself. Of course, you may have turned the clock back a while but you can't stop it. How fast it ticks on from this point will depend to a great degree on the level of protection you use from now on.

### spot check

**Latest is not always greatest. The laser may be the newest, and most talked about option for resurfacing, but you should not feel you are getting second best if your physician recommends a procedure other than laser peeling. If, for instance, you have slack skin over your jawline, surgery may be a better option, while for necks and chests, chemical peeling is usually preferable.**

## Case study 1

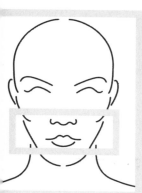

| | |
|---|---|
| Patient: | **Anna** |
| Age: | **In her 50s** |
| Problem: | **Upper lip wrinkles** |
| Procedure: | **Laser resurfacing** |
| Cost of treatment: | **£1250/$2000** |
| Result: | **Significant improvement lasting many years** |

### The dermatologist's story

This patient had moderate sun (photo) damage with some wrinkles on her top lip. We discussed a deep phenol peel but dismissed it as neither of us wanted to risk hypopigmentation. We looked at dermabrasion but rejected it on the grounds that the severe redness, risk of scarring and an uneven result were unacceptable for this part of the face and Anna's lifestyle.

We decided on the $CO_2$ laser because the healing time would be reduced and the device's precision meant that I could target specific lines as well as treat the whole area. I made two passes over her top lip which constituted a mid-depth peel and feathered the edges of the treated area to ensure the line between treated and untreated skin wasn't too marked.

It took eight days for her epidermis to regenerate, and during this time Anna was advised to cover her skin with gel dressings. Nowadays the treatment involves using gel dressings for the first 24 hours and then water soaks and moisturizers to keep the skin from drying out

Anna was treated five years ago and the results have held up well and she is still less lined on her upper lip than before.

### The patient's story

I've never smoked, nor sunbathed much being fair skinned, but I was living and working as a make-up artist in California and had developed four long deepish lines that ran from my lips almost to my nose, as well as some smaller more shallow ones. I had a 'phase one' laser peel. It really didn't hurt – just a series of tiny, quick burns. Actually, the smell was worse than the feeling. The whole thing took about ten minutes. Immediately afterwards my lip became a little swollen and purple, but I didn't need painkillers. In fact, I felt well enough to go out to dinner that night.

Over the next few days my top lip crusted; I looked as if I was wearing a strange fake moustache. I had to keep plying the scab with grease to keep it from cracking. But I went back to work almost immediately. Because this was California everyone was curious rather than judgemental. Many of my colleagues said they would be signing up for the procedure themselves. After five days the crust started peeling away and when it finally came off the skin underneath was smooth and clear. Five years later my lip is still perfect and now I'm going to have treatment on my eyes.

## Case study 2

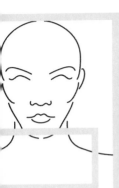

| | |
|---|---|
| Patient: | **Louisa** |
| Age: | **Late 50s** |
| Problem: | **Photo damage including sun spots (solar lentigo) to neck and chest** |
| Procedure: | **Medium TCA peel on neck and Jessner's peel on chest** |
| Cost of treatment: | **£800/$1280** |
| Result: | **Good improvement in pigmentation and tone lasting several years** |

### The dermatologist's story

Louise had moderate photo damage on her neck and more severe sun-related changes on her chest. Because the skin in these areas is thinner and less oily than facial skin it is more prone to heat damage. This is still sometimes a problem with laser treatment so we chose instead to treat the area with chemical peels. For her neck I used a 25 per cent TCA peel, and over her chest a Jessner's peel which would be more easily controlled by the dermatologist. The advantage of Jessner's is that you can paint on more layers as and when you see what the initial ones are doing. The procedure itself took just over an hour after which Louise went home with moisturizing creams to apply. A few days after the peels she returned complaining of burning and weeping of the wound which is unusual. I prescribed cortisone to alleviate the inflammation.

She kept in regular contact with the clinic so that we could monitor the healing process. After a somewhat prolonged healing phase we concluded there was a 50 per cent improvement in her skin quality.

### The patient's story

For 55 years I sunbathed as much as I could. I'd had dermabrasion over my face in 1971 but my neck and chest were covered in dark sun spots. The peel wasn't painful – over my neck I barely felt it. After two to three days, though, it began to weep and it felt as if it was on fire. I went back to the clinic and was given cortisone injections and gradually after two weeks the weeping and heat eased off.

Although there were times when I sorely doubted it, the final result was very good. I would say there is a 75–80 per cent improvement in general skin tone. I was spattered in brown spots and now there are only two left which we've talked about removing with the laser. It's a relief to have a chest that more closely matches my face. For years I wore high-necked dresses.

I also recently had my face treated with the laser. Again it really didn't hurt at all. My face was pretty red for a few weeks but I was amazed at how quickly and painlessly it healed. I'm very happy with the result.

# Q&A
## Questions & answers

**My child has eczema – I've read that hard water can exacerbate it. Should I install a water softener?**

It certainly can't harm and might help. We are not yet sure whether there is a direct or indirect link between childhood eczema and hard water. It may be that the alkaline salts themselves in hard water are causing or worsening the condition or that people in hard water areas tend to use more soap to get a lather. If you can't afford to install a water softener you should reduce your level of soap usage and not bother about getting a lather. Switch to non-soap cleansers such as Nutralia or Ph5.5 or try washing formulations made expressly for dermatological conditions (e.g. Dermol 500 lotion, Balnium, Oilatum, Wash 45).

**I have thread veins. What's the best method for getting rid of them?**

If they are very large they will have to be surgically removed. If small, the majority of upper legs veins are best treated by sclerotherapy. On the face and around the ankle, the laser should be used to avoid the risk of brain damage and blindness, or ulceration of leg arteries respectively. Where you have your veins treated is also important. I cringe at the thought of beauty salons doing it –

sclerotherapy carries the risk of anaphyaxsis, total shock shutdown which can kill. Ensure the person treating you has medical training, or at very least supervision (many dermatologists have their nurses perform sclerotherapy).

**Just how effective are lasers for hair removal?**

The long pulsed ruby lasers are proving to be very effective, normally permanently reducing 80 per cent of hair growth. Those with refrigerated wands carry the least risk of thermal damage or scarring. Your physician should always do a small test patch first. If you have olive skin and dark hair, you and your physician should proceed with caution as the laser can mistake skin pigment for hair colour and eradicate it. Fair skin and dark hair is the best combination for laser hair removal.

**Our local hospital has told us we shouldn't bother having our child's strawberry birthmark treated as it will probably go away of its own accord as she gets older. Is this true?**

Statistically, yes. Fifty per cent of strawberry hemangiomas have gone by the time the child is

5, 60 per cent by the age of 6, 70 per cent by 7. By ten, however, 10–20 per cent remain and even if the redness has gone, some slack skin may be left. There is now a growing feeling that it is wise to treat such birthmarks with pulsed dye vascular lasers because there is a better chance of total clearance and to avoid the risk of psychological damage that facial disfigurement often brings.

### Will I be more prone to sunburn while I'm using Retin A?

Yes, because your stratum corneum is thinner. A thick rough hide is a good sun block. It is therefore essential to apply daily sunscreen – not least because if you are using Retin-A to smooth your wrinkles you don't want further sun damage to cancel out its reparative work.

### If I stop using Retin-A or AHAs will my skin look worse than before?

No. It was thought that after stopping treatment your skin returned to its pre-treated state but there is increasing evidence to suggest that as long as you used, and continue to use, a daily sun-screening cream, some of the improvement you gained while on a cosmeceutical can be maintained. Instead of stopping altogether it can be useful to shift down to a 'maintenance regime' of applying Retin-A twice a week.

### Most of my wrinkles are around my eyes. Is it safe for me to apply my cosmeceutical here?

Yes, the thin skin in this area should normally tolerate very small amounts every second or third night and will usually show good improvement as a result. Remember to remove all your eye-make-up and wash your face very gently before applying it.

### How do I know how long my temporary filler will last?

Unfortunately, there is no way of predicting exactly how long a substance will last in any individual as it will depend on the site and the amount of sun damage to your skin. However, your physician should be able to give you a fair idea, to within two or three months.

### What if I simply don't like the look of my injection or implant?

The temporary fillers will gradually be reabsorbed but you will have to wait from three to twelve months for this to happen. Softform can be easily removed at any time. However, if you have opted for other permanent fillers you do have a problem. Silicone and Artecol cannot be taken out and Gortex can be, but with difficulty, and often not without some tissue damage.

### I am Asian and have very dark skin. Am I a suitable for a peel?

With any resurfacing procedure there is a risk of the patient developing unevenly pigmented areas. However, the more deeply pigmented your skin, the greater the risk, so dark Mediterranean, Asian and black patients should be fully appraised of the risks before signing up for such a procedure. That said, the new lasers are so extraordinarily accurate that the chance of an uneven result is greatly lessened.

### I'm considering a face lift and a peel. Which should I have first?

My advice would be to have a peel first and then decide whether you still need surgery. Particularly with the laser, there is a good degree of collagen fibre shrinkage which results in a tightening, lifting effect. If you later decide you still want surgery, your improved complexion will not be affected.

# index

# picture credits

# bibliography

ABC of Dermatology 3rd edition PK Buxton, (BMJ Publishing, London, 1998)

Retinoids – A Clinician's Guide 2nd edition Nicholas J Lowe & Ronald Marks, Retinoids (Martin Dunitz, London, England 1998

Cosmetics in Dermatology 2nd edition Zoe Diana Draelos (Churchill Livingston, New York, 1995)

Cutaneous Medicine and Surgery KA Arndt, PE Leboit, JK Robinson, BU Wintroub, (WB Saunders, Philadelphia, Penn 1996)

Sunscreens – Development, Evaluation, and Regulatory Aspects 2nd edition Nicholas J Lowe, Nadim A Shaath, Madhu A Pathak editors Sunscreens (Marcel Dekker, New York 1997)

Hair and Scalp Disorders Rodney Dawber, Dominique Van Neste (Martin Dunitz, London 1995

Photodamage Barbara Gilchrest (Blackwell Science, Cambridge Mass. 1995)

A Text Atlas of Nail Disorders Robert Baran, Rodney Dawber, Eckart Haneke, Antonella Tosti (Martin Dunitz, London 1996)

Textbook of Cosmetic Dermatology 2nd edition R Baran, HI Maibach, editors (Martin Dunitz, London, 1998

Textbook of Dermatology 5th edition A Rook, DS Wilkinson, FJG Ebling, RH Champion, JL Burton, (Blackwell Scientific Publications, 1994)